Baillière's

CLINICAL PAEDIATRICS

INTERNATIONAL PRACTICE AND RESEARCH

Baillière's

CLINICAL PAEDIATRICS

INTERNATIONAL PRACTICE AND RESEARCH

Volume 3/Number 4
November 1995

Leukaemia and Lymphoma

J. M. CHESSELLS
I. M. HANN
Guest Editors

Baillière Tindall
London Philadelphia Sydney Tokyo Toronto

This book is printed on acid-free paper.

Baillière Tindall
W. B. Saunders
Company Ltd

24–28 Oval Road,
London NW1 7DX

The Curtis Center, Independence Square West,
Philadelphia, PA 19106–3399, USA

55 Horner Avenue
Toronto, Ontario M8Z 4X6, Canada

Harcourt Brace & Company
Australia
30–52 Smidmore Street, Marrickville, NSW 2204, Australia

Harcourt Brace & Company
Japan Inc,
Ichibancho Central Building, 22–1
Ichibancho, Chiyoda-ku, Tokyo 102, Japan

ISSN 0963–6714

ISBN 0–7020–2075–3 (single copy)

Baillière's Clinical Paediatrics is published four times each year by Baillière Tindall. Prices for Volume 3 (1995) are:

TERRITORY	ANNUAL SUBSCRIPTION	SINGLE ISSUE
Europe including UK	£86.00 (Institutional) post free £74.00 (Individual) post free	£30.00 post free
All other countries	Consult your local Harcourt Brace & Company office for dollar price	

The editor of this publication is Gail Greensmith, Baillière Tindall, 24–28 Oval Road, London NW1 7DX.

Typeset by Phoenix Photosetting, Chatham.
Printed and bound in Great Britain by the University Printing House, Cambridge.

Contributors to this issue

RICHARD L. CARTER MA, DM, DSc, FRCPath, FFPM, Honorary Consultant Histopathologist, Royal Marsden Hospital, Department of Paediatrics, Downs Road, Sutton, Surrey SM2 5PT, UK; and Professorial Research Fellow, Robens Institute, University of Surrey, UK.

JUDITH M. CHESSELLS MBBS, MD, FRCP, DObst, RCOG, FRCPath, Professor in Haematology/Oncology, Great Ormond Street Hospital for Children NHS Trust, London WC1N 3JH, UK.

ANN GOLDMAN MA, MB, FRCP, Clinical Consultant in Palliative Care, Great Ormond Street Hospital for Children NHS Trust, London WC1N 3JH, UK; and Honorary Senior Lecturer, Institute of Child Health, Guildford Street, London, UK.

IAN M. HANN MD, FRCP, FRCPath, Consultant Haematologist and Honorary Senior Lecturer, Great Ormond Street Hospital for Children NHS Trust, London WC1N 3JH, UK.

MERIEL E. M. JENNEY MD, MRCP, Consultant Paediatric Oncologist, Department of Haematology and Oncology, Royal Manchester Children's Hospital, Pendlebury, Manchester M27 4HA, UK.

GEORGE D. N. KISSEN BSc, MBChB, DCH, General Practitioner, Stretford, Manchester; and Hospital Practitioner, Manchester Children's Hospital, Department of Haematology and Oncology, Pendlebury, Manchester M27 4HA, UK.

SVERRE O. LIE MD, PhD, Professor and CHairman, Department of Pediatrics, Rikshospitalet, University Hospital, 0027 Oslo, Norway.

JOHN S. LILLEYMAN FRCP, FRCPath, Professor of Paediatric Oncology, St Bartholomew's Hospital Medical College, West Smithfield, London EC1A 7BE, UK.

KEITH P. McCARTHY MD, MRCPath, Consultant Histopathologist, Royal Marsden Hospital, Fulham Road, London SW6 6JT, UK.

CATHERINE PATTE MD, Institut Gustave Roussy, Department of Paediatric Oncology/Haematology, 11, Rue Camille Desmoulins, 94805 Villejuif, France.

KENT A. ROBERTSON MD, PhD, FAAP, Assistant Professor of Pediatrics, James Whitcomb Riley Hospital for Children, Indiana University Medical Center, 702 Barnhill Drive, Indianapolis IN 46202-5225, USA.

LESLIE L. ROBISON PhD, Professor of Pediatrics and Director, Division of Pediatric Epidemiology and Clinical Research, University of Minnesota, 420 Delaware Street SE, Box 422, Minneapolis MN 55455, USA.

TOM R. ROGERS MA, MSc, FRCPath, FRCPI, Professor of Infectious Diseases and Bacteriology, Department of Infectious Diseases and Bacteriology, Royal Postgraduate Medical School, Ducane Road, Hammersmith, London W12 0NN, UK.

JULIE A. ROSS PhD, University of Minnesota, Division Pediatric Epidemiology/Clinical Research, PO Box 422 U.M.H.C., Minneapolis MN 55455, USA.

FRANKLIN O. SMITH MD, FAAP, Associate Professor of Pediatrics, James Whitcomb Riley Hospital for Children, Indiana University Medical Center, 702 Barnhill Drive, Indianapolis IN 46202-5225, USA.

Table of contents

PREVIOUS ISSUE

Vol. 1, No. 3 1993
Arthritis in Children and Adolescents
T. R. Southwood & P. N. Malleson

Vol. 1, No. 4 1993
Transplantation
M. Broyer

Vol. 2, No. 1 1994
Coma
J. A. Eyre

Vol. 2, No. 2 1994
Current Issues in the Adolescent Patient
R. S. Tonkin

Vol. 2, No. 3 1994
Epilepsy
E. M. Ross & R. C. Woody

Vol. 2, No. 4 1994
Paediatric Gastroenterology
B. S. Kirschner & J. A. Walker-Smith

Vol. 3, No. 1 1995
Pulmonary Problems in the Perinatal Period and their Sequelae
V. Y. H. Yu

Vol. 3, No. 2 1995
Asthma
P. D. Phelan

Vol. 3, No. 3 1995
Stress and Pain in Infancy and Childhood
A. Aynsley-Green, M. P. Ward Platt & A. R. Lloyd-Thomas

FORTHCOMING ISSUE

Vol. 4, No. 1 1996
Cardiology for General Paediatricians
B. W. McCrindle

Preface

Leukaemias and lymphomas account for over 40% of cancers in childhood. They have clinical, epidemiological and pathological similarities and all are primarily chemocurable; thus justifying a combined volume about recent advances in management. We aim in this issue of *Baillière's Clinical Paediatrics* to cover both the general treatment topics of most relevance to paediatricians and to provide an overview of recent specific therapeutic advances.

Few paediatricians can be unaware of the recent interest in epidemiology of these disorders, now a subject of several national studies. Advances in immunology, cytogenetics and molecular biology have improved the classification of all lymphoproliferative malignancies and have produced a more rational approach to treatment, particularly for the non-Hodgkin lymphomas. For the general paediatrician involved in shared care, the issues of family and supportive care and management of infectious complications of treatment are clearly important. There is now an increasing population of children who have been cured of cancer and leukaemia, and optimizing appropriate and sensitive follow-up of such patients is a major challenge for us all.

The authors have also reviewed modern developments in therapy, and have been asked to emphasize principles of treatment rather than ever changing protocols. Perhaps here, one of the most encouraging results is the improved outcome for children with the rarer myeloid type of acute leukaemia, hitherto a uniformly fatal disease; but steady advances have been made in treatment of all leukaemias and lymphomas. No book on this topic would be complete without a review of the role of high dose chemo/radiotherapy and transfusion of stem cells, whether autologous, allogeneic or unrelated, and the authors have attempted to put this therapy into perspective.

As the authorship of this volume shows, advances in management come from collaboration between specialists in all disciplines, both national and international.

JUDITH CHESSELLS
IAN HANN

1

Epidemiology of leukaemias and lymphomas in childhood

LESLIE L. ROBISON
JULIE A. ROSS

In North America and western Europe, leukaemia and lymphoma represent approximately 40% of cancers that occur in the paediatric age group, although this distribution differs substantially in selected regions around the world (Parkin et al, 1988). Because acute lymphoblastic leukaemia (ALL) represents the most common form of childhood cancer, it is not surprising that, over the years, ALL has been the focus of a relatively large number of epidemiological investigations. In contrast, because of the relative rarity of non-Hodgkin's lymphoma and Hodgkin's disease, these tumours have been studied less extensively.

Presented in this chapter is an overview of selected epidemiological characteristics of childhood acute leukaemia, non-Hodgkin's lymphoma and Hodgkin's disease. The intent is to provide a reasonable description of the features generally agreed to be characteristic of these groups of diseases, while providing a context within which to evaluate the aetiological importance of known or suggested risk factors.

ACUTE LYMPHOBLASTIC LEUKAEMIA

Classification

Acute lymphoblastic leukaemia (ALL) is a heterogeneous disease; both immunological and morphological classifications exist (Henderson and Lister, 1990). Immunological classifications, which use cell-surface proteins of the malignant cells, include T-cell and B-cell leukaemia. B-cell leukaemia is further subdivided, depending on the degree of differentiation of the cell of origin. Morphological classifications, based on the French–American–British (FAB) system, include L1, L2 and L3 (Henderson and Lister, 1990). Clinicians use these classifications when considering therapy, as patients can be at varying degrees of risk of relapse depending on the type of ALL. With a few exceptions (Greaves et al, 1993; Buckley et al, 1994), however, the disease has been treated as one entity in

Baillière's Clinical Paediatrics—
Vol. 3, No. 4, November 1995
ISBN 0–7020–2075–3

epidemiological studies. This is due primarily to the large number of cases needed to assess the magnitude of a specific risk factor and the relative lack of uniformity in classification. As there is evidence that the incidence of ALL in specific subclasses is not consistent geographically (Greaves et al, 1993), large studies are currently being conducted that should have sufficient power to test specific hypotheses among subgroups.

Incidence

Significant international variations exist in the incidence of childhood ALL, with rates ranging from 9 per million to 47 per million for males, and from 7 per million to 43 per million for females (Parkin et al, 1988). Figure 1 depicts incidence rates of ALL for selected countries. Notably, incidence rates are highest in the USA (among whites) and in Australia (New South Wales), Costa Rica and the Federal Republic of Germany (the former 'West Germany'). Intermediate rates exist in most European countries, while the lowest rates of ALL occur in American blacks and in India (Bombay) and Kuwait. For most countries, the incidence of ALL is higher in males. However, some notable exceptions include Kuwait (where the rate ratio of females:males is 1.2) and American blacks (rate ratio approximately 1.0).

Figure 2 illustrates ALL age-specific incidence rates for children diagnosed below 15 years of age using the United States Surveillance Epidemiology and End Results (SEER) programme data. Overall, there is

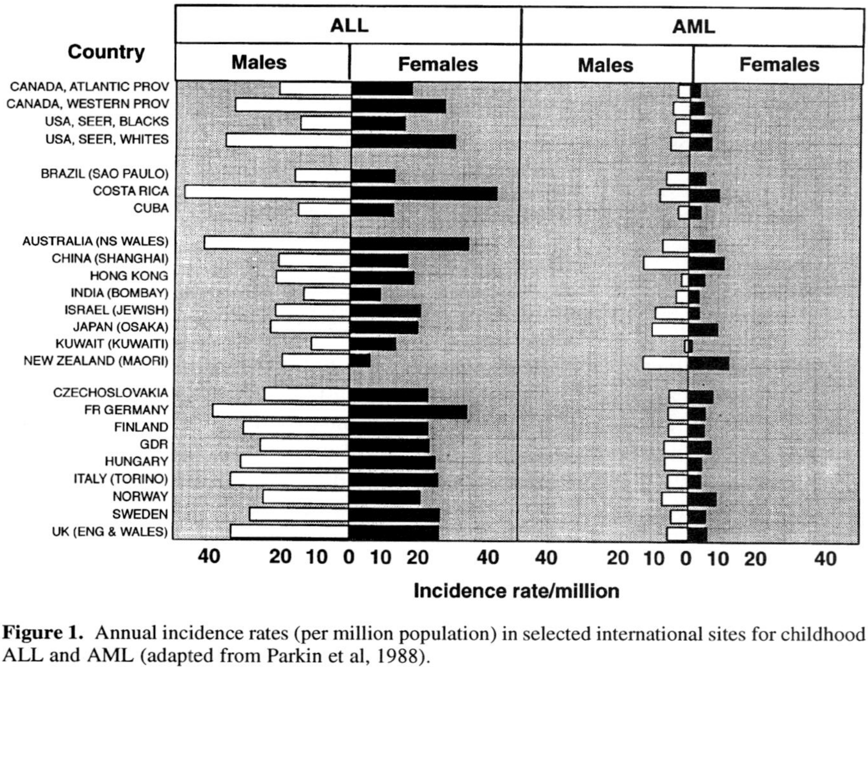

Figure 1. Annual incidence rates (per million population) in selected international sites for childhood ALL and AML (adapted from Parkin et al, 1988).

a significant peak in incidence that occurs between 3 and 5 years of age. This peak did not appear until the 1930s in children living in the United States and Great Britain (Court-Brown and Doll, 1961) and it is notably absent in many developing countries (reviewed in Ross et al, 1994). This has led some to theorize that exposures associated with modernization may lead to leukaemia (Ramot and Magrath, 1982). The incidence in males is marginally higher than in females with two notable exceptions: (1) infant leukaemia, where there is a female predominance, and (2) T-cell ALL, where the male : female ratio is approximately 4 : 1 (Kersey et al, 1973). Finally, for younger ages, the incidence in whites is approximately two-fold higher than in blacks. It is unknown what would account for this marked difference between the races; however, it is peculiar that the young age peak in incidence did not appear in blacks until the 1960s (Pierce et al, 1969).

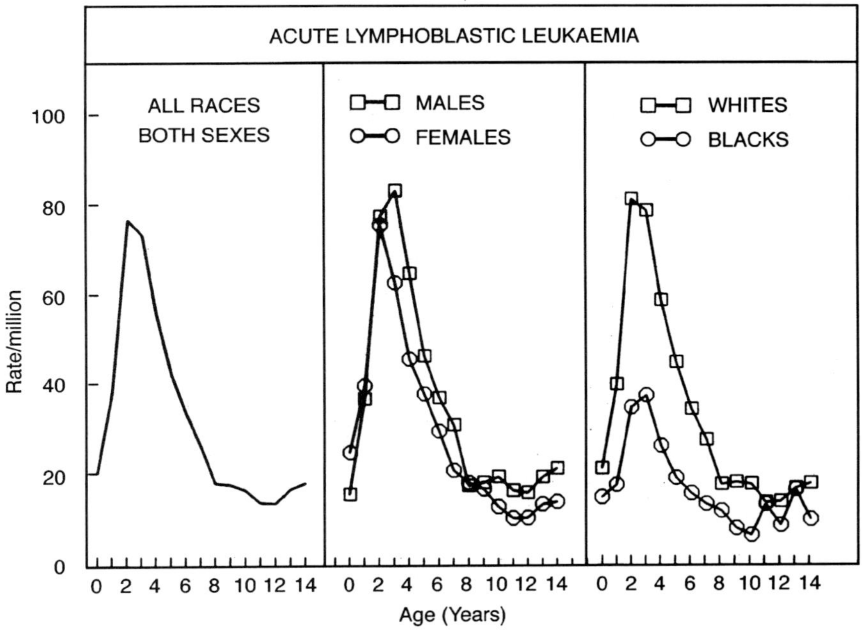

Figure 2. Age-, gender-, and race-specific annual incidence rates (per million population) for acute lymphoblastic leukaemia in children in the USA under the age of 15 years (adapted from Gurney et al, 1995).

Genetic associations

A number of genetic syndromes have been associated with an increased risk of childhood leukaemia, although they account for a small proportion of cases (Table 1). The most striking association is between Down syndrome and both ALL and acute myeloid leukaemia (AML). Approximately 2% of children diagnosed with ALL or AML have Down syndrome, representing an approximate 12-fold higher risk of leukaemia than the general population (Robison and Neglia, 1987). An increased risk of ALL has also been associated with neurofibromatosis (Bader and Miller, 1978), Shwachman syndrome (Woods et al, 1981), Bloom syndrome (German et al, 1979), ataxia telangiectasia (Hecht and Hecht, 1990), Langerhans cell histiocytosis (Arico et al, 1993) and Klinefelter's syndrome (Shaw et al, 1992).

Acquired genetic abnormalities have also been reported in ALL (Table 1). A few cases of ALL have demonstrated the Philadelphia chromosome translocation t(9;22) (Crist et al, 1990). Moreover, a specific subtype of ALL has been associated with t(1;19) (Secker-Walker et al, 1992). B-cell ALL (Burkitt lymphoma) and certain T-cell ALL have been associated with specific abnormalities (Henderson and Lister, 1990; Kennedy et al, 1991). However, except for infant leukaemia (both ALL and AML), in which approximately 80% of cases appear to have an abnormality involving chromosome band 11q23 (Cimino et al, 1993), there do not appear to be any consistent genetic abnormalities that are associated with childhood ALL.

Table 1. Genetic syndromes and chromosomal abnormalities association with childhood acute leukaemia.

Syndrome or chromosomal abnormality	Childhood leukaemia type	Comment
Down syndrome	ALL and AML	Most striking association; approximately 12-fold higher risk of leukaemia in children with Down syndrome
Neurofibromatosis	ALL and AML	Higher proportion of leukaemia cases are AML rather than ALL
Ataxia telangiectasia	ALL and AML	
(Klinefelter syndrome)*	ALL	Report of two cases
(Langerhans cell histiocytosis)	ALL	Report of two cases
(Bloom syndrome)	ALL and AML	Report of six childhood cases
(Shwachman syndrome)	ALL and AML	Compilation of seven case reports
Familial monosomy 7	AML	Familial form is where two or more siblings develop MPS† or AML before 20; possibly involves a tumour suppressor gene
(Kostmann granulocytopenia)	AML	Report of two cases
Fanconi anaemia	AML	

* Report in parentheses based on a few cases noted in the literature.
† Myeloproliferative syndrome.

The first observations of familial leukaemia were published four decades ago, when it was noted that clusters of leukaemia had occurred across generations of certain families (Anderson, 1955). Since that time, similar leukaemia families have been reported in the literature (reviewed in Linet, 1985). There is also evidence that leukaemias can cluster in families that experience a high frequency of other cancers, including brain tumours, colon cancer, and stomach cancer (Maklin, 1960; Farwell and Flannery, 1984). Familial case reports can be informative and may provide clues about aetiology, although they are not representative of the majority of childhood leukaemias. Although these observations could suggest a genetic component to the aetiology, they may also reflect a shared environmental exposure. Some intriguing associations have also come from twin studies of leukaemia. Not only does there appear to be a high degree of concordance of leukaemia among twins (particularly monozygotic), but the risk of leukaemia is dependent on age, being elevated most in infants (reviewed in Strong, 1984). Some reports have suggested a risk that approaches 100% for the unaffected twin sibling of a monozygotic twin diagnosed at less than 1 year of age (Strong, 1984). In these cases, concordance may be due to shared placental circulation that allows the transfer of leukaemia cells from one twin to the other, and there exists some molecular evidence to support this theory (Ford et al, 1993).

Demographic and environmental risk factors

The vast majority of epidemiological investigations of childhood leukaemia have utilized the case–control approach. This methodology involves the identification and comparison of specific characteristics of cases and a selected population of controls (those without the disease of interest). Since case–control studies generally do not provide direct evidence of causation, they are used primarily in conjunction with other scientific data in order better to understand the aetiology.

Table 2 summarizes many of the factors (both demographic and environmental) that have been examined in relation to risk of childhood ALL. By and large, there have been consistent reports of an increased risk of ALL in the individuals of middle and upper socio-economic status (SES) (reviewed in Ross et al, 1994). SES as a individual risk factor for childhood ALL is difficult to intepret as it may represent a myriad of factors, including life style, location of residence, parental occupation, maternal age, etc. An increased risk of childhood ALL has been consistently observed to be associated with high birth-weight, although there have been a few exceptions (reviewed in Ross et al, 1994). In particular, the positive association with birth-weight has been confined to children diagnosed at younger ages. Moreover, similar increased risks have been observed in other childhood cancers, including neuroblastoma, astrocytoma, and Wilms' tumour (Ross et al, 1994; Leisenring et al, 1994). At present, it is unknown why high birth-weight confers a greater risk of certain childhood cancers; however, there is some speculation that growth factors may be involved in some instances (Olshan, 1986).

Several investigators have examined maternal reproductive history as a risk factor for ALL (reviewed in Ross et al, 1994). With one exception (Shu et al, 1988), these studies have found an increased risk of ALL with prior history of fetal loss, with elevated risks ranging in magnitude from 2–5 times higher than when no previous fetal loss had been reported. Furthermore, in the most recent study to date (Yeazel et al, 1995), the investigators not only found the association to be present in ALL cases diagnosed in the first several years of life, but also noted a significant trend with increasing numbers of fetal loss (report of one fetal loss increased the

Table 2. Selected descriptive, demographic and environmental variables examined in childhood ALL.

	Variable	Specifics	Comment
Descriptive	Sex	Male > female	Approximately 1.3 fold higher risk
	Age		Peak in incidence between ages 3 and 5
	Race	White > black	Approximately 2-fold higher risk
Demographic	Socio-economic status	Middle and upper SES classes	Increased risk; fairly consistent
	Birth-weight	> 4000 grams (> 3500 grams, Shanghai)	Approximately 2-fold increased risk; fairly consistent
	Maternal reproductive history	Fetal loss prior to index child's birth	Approximately 2–5 fold increased risk; fairly consistent
	(Maternal age)*	Age > 35 at pregnancy	Slight increased risk; somewhat inconsistent
	(Birth order)	First born	Some studies have reported a slight increased risk; inconsistent, may be surrogate measure for timing of exposure to infectious agents
Environmental	Radiation	Prenatal exposure	Increased risk; consistent, but now accounts for very few cases
	Radiation	Postnatal diagnostic	No increased risk
	Radiation	Postnatal therapeutic	Increased risk
	(Radiation)	Paternal exposure	Inconsistent; further investigation is warranted
	(Electromagnetic fields)	Children living near high voltage EMF	Inconsistent; large studies in four countries are currently in progress
	(Smoking)	Maternal smoking during pregnancy	Inconsistent
	(Alcohol)	Maternal drinking during pregnancy	No association in two studies
	(Pesticides)	Parental exposure around the time of pregnancy	Increased risk noted in a few studies; biological plausibility is high; subject of several current studies
	(Occupations)	Parental	Isolated reports of an increased risk with motor vehicle exhaust, hydrocarbons, solvents, paints; subject of several current studies
	(Postnatal infection)		Inconsistent; however, subject of at least two hypotheses; further integration of molecular biology and epidemiology will help answer this question
	(Vitamin K)	Intramuscular neonatal administration	Increased risk first reported in the 1990s (leukaemia type not specified); more recent studies have found no association; unlikely to be a major risk factor for leukaemia
	(Diet)	Child's consumption of hot dogs, cod liver oil, etc.	These associations (either as increased or decreased risk) may be due to chance; a large-scale study investigating childhood leukaemia (ALL and AML) and diet is needed

*Risk factors in parentheses indicate either inconsistent findings or risk not yet extensively evaluated. The majority of these variables have been recently reviewed (Ross et al, 1994).

risk five-fold, while report of two or more previous losses increased the risk 25-fold). Fetal loss may represent an indicator of genetic predisposition and/or chronic environmental exposure. An increased risk of ALL has also been associated with advanced maternal age, even after adjustment for Down syndrome. Although this association has not been uniformly consistent across studies, in general the risk increases after the age of 35 years (Ross et al, 1994).

Additional studies have examined maternal smoking and drinking during the pregnancy of the index child and subsequent risk of leukaemia. Several studies have identified an elevated risk of ALL with maternal smoking, while others have found no association (Ross et al, 1994). Two studies have reported negative associations with maternal alcohol consumption, one that examined ALL specifically and the other that examined all leukaemias combined (van Steensel-Moll et al, 1985; McKinney et al, 1987).

Environmental influences have been examined with respect to childhood ALL, particularly as more knowledge has been gained from the study of adult leukaemia. Perhaps the most comprehensively studied environmental risk factor for ALL has been in utero exposure to diagnostic ionizing radiation. Stewart et al (1958) first reported an increased risk of childhood leukaemia associated with prenatal exposure to X-rays. Since that time, several studies have confirmed this finding (Ross et al, 1994). Relative risks range in magnitude from 1.5- to 1.7-fold. In utero exposure to diagnostic radiation is generally considered to be an established risk factor for childhood leukaemia (both ALL and AML), albeit accounting for a very small proportion of cases.

Children who receive radiation therapy for the treatment of Hodgkin's disease, Langerhans cell histiocytosis, thymus enlargement, and tinea capitis also appear to have a slightly elevated risk of leukaemia, whereas postnatal *diagnostic* radiation is not considered to be a risk factor for ALL (Ross et al, 1994). However, persons exposed to the atomic bomb blasts in Hiroshima and Nagasaki as children were found to be at an increased risk of both ALL and AML (Jablon et al, 1971; Preston et al, 1994).

Paternal preconception exposure to radiation has been the subject of several recent investigations. In Great Britain, an eight-fold higher risk of childhood leukaemia was reported in fathers preconceptionally exposed to high levels of radiation in a nuclear power plant (Gardner, 1991). However, a similar study in Canada found no elevated risk of leukaemia in offspring (McLaughlin et al, 1993). More recently, a study in the USA found an elevated risk of ALL in children whose fathers were preconceptionally exposed to diagnostic X-rays, with a statistically significant three-fold increased risk being associated with X-rays of the lower abdomen (Shu et al, 1994). The biological plausibility for an association between paternal preconception radiation exposure and leukaemia is controversial (Doll et al, 1994); future identification of molecular markers will help to determine whether these associations are real or due to chance.

Exposure to electromagnetic fields has been investigated in a number of studies, motivated in part by the ubiquitousness of the exposure, epidemiological studies suggesting an association, and data from laboratory studies indicating that adverse biological effects may occur (reviewed in Stevens, 1993). An elevated risk of childhood ALL among children living in close proximity to high-current-carrying-capacity electric wires was first reported by Wertheimer and Leeper (1979); these findings were later confirmed by Savitz et al (1988). Since that time, a number of studies have been conducted exploring these associations; some have reported an elevated risk, while others have found no association (Ross et al, 1994). There are methodological problems in measuring exposure to electromagnetic fields, and there is the potential for confounding from other variables (including city-versus-rural living, race and socio-economic status). A number of countries are currently conducting large case–control studies to explore these associations.

Parental occupations have also been examined in a number of studies. Increased risk of ALL in offspring has been reported to be associated with parental occupational exposure to solvents, hydrocarbons or paints (reviewed in Ross et al, 1994). In one study, exposure to motor vehicle exhaust was associated with an increased risk of infant ALL (Vianna et al, 1984). Elevated risk of ALL has also been noted with parental exposure to pesticides. Many pesticides contain organophosphates, which, in animal studies, have been associated with leukaemia in the young (Gibel and Lohs, 1975). Large studies are currently underway to assess parental occupation and pesticide exposure in both childhood ALL and AML.

Other exposures that have recently been of interest include intramuscular vitamin K exposure (Golding et al, 1992), chloramphenicol use in offspring (Shu et al, 1987), and diet of either parents or the index child (Shu et al, 1988; Peters et al, 1994). Based on recent findings from studies in the United States and Sweden, intramuscular vitamin K is unlikely to be a risk factor for childhood ALL (Klebanoff et al, 1993; Ekelund et al, 1993). On the other hand, diet has not been extensively investigated in either childhood ALL or AML; however, diet does appear to be important in childhood brain tumours (Bunin et al, 1993).

Finally, viral infections have been associated with certain human cancers, including T-cell leukaemia and African Burkitt lymphoma (Cotran et al, 1989). There was an early report suggesting an increase in childhood ALL following an outbreak of influenza (Austin et al, 1975), but this finding has not been reproduced. An association between exposure to viral agents and childhood ALL has not been documented, although there has been speculation that feline leukaemia virus or bovine leukaemia virus may be important in the aetiology (reviewed in Ross et al, 1994). In attempting to explain the peak in ALL incidence occurring between the ages of 3 and 5, Greaves (1988) proposed a theory suggesting that early exposure to infection may be protective toward the development of childhood leukaemia. In fact, associations with birth-order and socio-economic status might be partly explained by delayed exposure to infectious agents (due either to fewer siblings or to delayed entry into daycare (James, 1990)).

ACUTE MYELOID LEUKAEMIA

Classification

Like ALL, acute myeloid leukaemia (AML) is a heterogeneous group of diseases. Eight distinct morphological classifications exist for AML, including M0 (myeloid leukaemia with minimal differentiation), M1 (acute myeloblastic—undifferentiated), M2 (acute myeloblastic—differentiated), M3 (acute promyelocytic), M4 (acute myelomonocytic), M5 (acute monocytic), M6 (acute erythroblastic) and M7 (acute megakaryoblastic) (Henderson and Lister, 1990; Creutzig et al, 1993). Childhood AML is most often found as AML-M2, AML-M4 and AML-M5, although there are distinctions depending on the age of diagnosis.

Incidence

As with ALL, significant international variations in incidence exist with AML. Shown in Figure 1, incidence rates of AML range from about 1 per million to 14 per million for males and from 1 per million to 10 per million for females (Parkin et al, 1988). AML rates are highest in Shanghai, Japan and in the New Zealand Maori people. Intermediate rates exist in Australia, the United States and the United Kingdom. The lowest rates occur in Kuwait and India. It should be noted that the higher incidence rate of AML in Shanghai is in contrast to the low incidence of ALL (Tu and Li, 1983). Unlike ALL, there is an approximately 1:1 ratio in the overall incidence rates of males:females.

AML incidence rates in children under the age of 15 using SEER data are depicted in Figure 3. Unlike ALL, there is no striking age peak in AML; however, there appears to be an elevated incidence in the very young. Except for infants, where there is a female predominance, there is no marked variation in incidence rates between the sexes in childhood AML. Finally, the incidence of AML is approximately two-fold higher in whites versus blacks under the age of 2; thereafter the incidence rates are quite similar. Although not shown, SEER data indicate that incidence rates are particularly high in Los Angeles Hispanics, with rates approaching 9 per million (Parkin et al, 1988).

Genetic associations

Similar to ALL, there are a number of genetic syndromes associated with childhood AML, including Down syndrome (Table 1). The AML morphological type most often associated with Down syndrome is AML-M7, with the estimated incidence of AML-M7 in children with Down syndrome being approximately 500 times that of normal children (Zipursky et al, 1987). For children with neurofibromatosis who subsequently develop leukaemia, there is a much higher proportion of cases with AML than ALL (Bader and Miller, 1978). There are a number of chromosomal abnormalities associated specifically with AML including inv(16) (LeBeau et al,

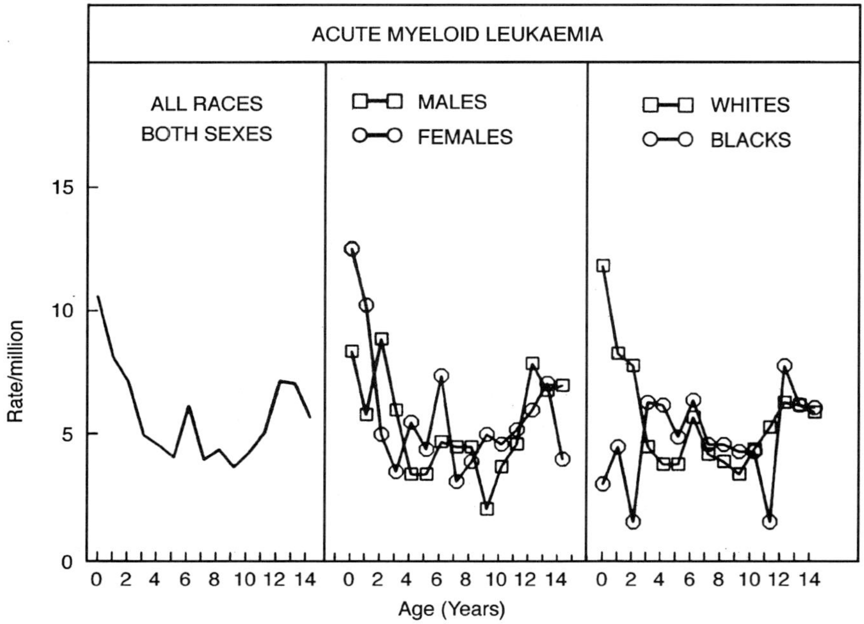

Figure 3. Age-, gender-, and race-specific annual incidence rates (per million population) for acute myeloid leukaemia in children in the USA under the age of 15 years (adapted from Gurney et al, 1995).

1983), trisomy 8 and t(8;21) (Woods et al, 1985) and t(15;17) (Stone and Mayer, 1990). Loss of chromosome 5 and or 7 is also associated with AML, particularly in secondary cases that occur as the result of cytotoxic chemotherapy regimens (LeBeau et al, 1986). Point mutations involving specific ras genes have also been associated with childhood AML (Volgelstein et al, 1990). Finally, like ALL, translocations involving the gene at chromosome band 11q23 occur frequently in infant AML (Cimino et al, 1993). Intriguingly, similar abnormalities at 11q23 have been observed in secondary AML cases occurring as the result of chemotherapy regimens that include epipodophyllotoxins (Pui et al, 1991).

Demographic and environmental risk factors

A number of studies conducted in *adult* AML have reported increased risks associated with specific occupations, including benzene worker, petrol station attendant, oil refinery worker, farmer and rubber worker (reviewed in Linet, 1985). Moreover, increased risks of adult AML have been associated with smoking (Siegel, 1993). Ecological studies have shown an increased incidence of adult and childhood AML in areas that have high levels of radon (Eatough and Henshaw, 1993; Viel, 1993). Based on results from studies of adult AML, a number of analytical studies have been initiated for childhood AML to explore potential relationships. Of the few studies completed to date (Table 3), the findings are summarized below.

For maternal reproductive history, findings in AML are similar to those reported for ALL (Yeazel et al, 1995). For AML cases diagnosed before 2 years of age, one previous fetal loss was associated with a five-fold increased risk, while two or more losses were associated with a 12-fold increased risk.

Two studies have reported an increased risk of AML (approximately two-fold) with maternal alcohol consumption during pregnancy (Severson et al, 1993; van Duijn et al, 1994); however, no increased risk of AML has been found with maternal smoking. One study reported an 11-fold increased risk of AML associated with maternal illicit drug use (primarily marijuana) during the index pregnancy (Robison et al, 1989). This same study also found a two-fold increased risk with maternal use of anti-nausea medications. As observed in childhood ALL, Shu et al (1987) reported that postnatal use of chloramphenicol was associated with an increased risk of childhood AML.

Parental occupational exposures have been explored in a few studies. In a study of 204 cases of childhood AML, parental pesticide exposure was associated with an 11-fold higher risk in children diagnosed under 6 years of age (Buckley et al, 1989). Moreover, the association was most apparent in cases with AML-M4 and AML-M5 who, characteristic of these morphology groups, were younger at the time of diagnosis. In this same study, paternal exposures to solvents, plastics, petroleum products, or lead were also associated with an increased risk. Shu et al (1988) found that maternal exposure to benzene or gasoline was associated with an increased risk of childhood AML. Several relatively large epidemiological studies examining parental and child exposure to pesticides, solvents, hydrocarbons, paints, etc. and subsequent risk of childhood AML are currently in progress; they should be able to provide further evidence for or against aetiological associations.

NON-HODGKIN'S LYMPHOMA

Incidence

Non-Hodgkin's lymphoma (NHL) accounts for approximately 6% of childhood cancer in the United States (Gurney et al, 1995). In the 0–19 age range, the incidence of NHL in the USA has been reported to be increasing at an average annual rate of approximately 1.4%; most of this increase appears to be within the 15–19 year age group (Miller et al, 1993). Changes in the classification of NHL have resulted in some difficulties in the interpretation of secular trends, particularly on an international basis (Banks, 1992). Internationally, there are remarkable differences in the incidence of NHL (Figure 4). In regions of Africa, the incidence of lymphoma (Hodgkin's and non-Hodgkin's) is approximately three times higher than

Table 3. Selected descriptive, demographic and environmental variables examined in childhood AML.

	Variable	Specifics	Comment
Descriptive	Sex	Male = female	
	Age		Incidence rates relatively constant to the age of 20
	Race	Hispanic	Highest rates reported in Los Angeles Hispanics
Demographic	(Maternal reproductive history)*	Fetal loss prior to the index child	One recent study has reported an increased risk similar to that seen with ALL
	Radiation	Prenatal exposure	Consistent, but now accounts for very few cases
Environmental	(Pesticides)	Parental exposure	As in ALL, increased risk noted; coincides with data on adult AML; also subject of several current studies
	(Benzene)	Paternal exposure	Somewhat inconsistent, although magnitude of risk about 4–5-fold
	(Smoking)	Maternal smoking during pregnancy	Little evidence of an increased risk
	(Alcohol)	Maternal drinking during pregnancy	Two recent studies have reported an elevated risk; further investigation is warranted
	(Drug and medication use)	Marijuana, morning sickness medication, others	Isolated studies have reported an elevated risk of AML with maternal marijuana-use (11-fold) and anti-nausea medication (3-fold). Also, chloramphenicol (child) use was associated with elevated risks of both AML and ALL; further study is warranted

* Risk factors in parentheses indicate either inconsistent findings or risk not yet extensively evaluated. The majority of these variables have been recently reviewed (Ross et al, 1994).

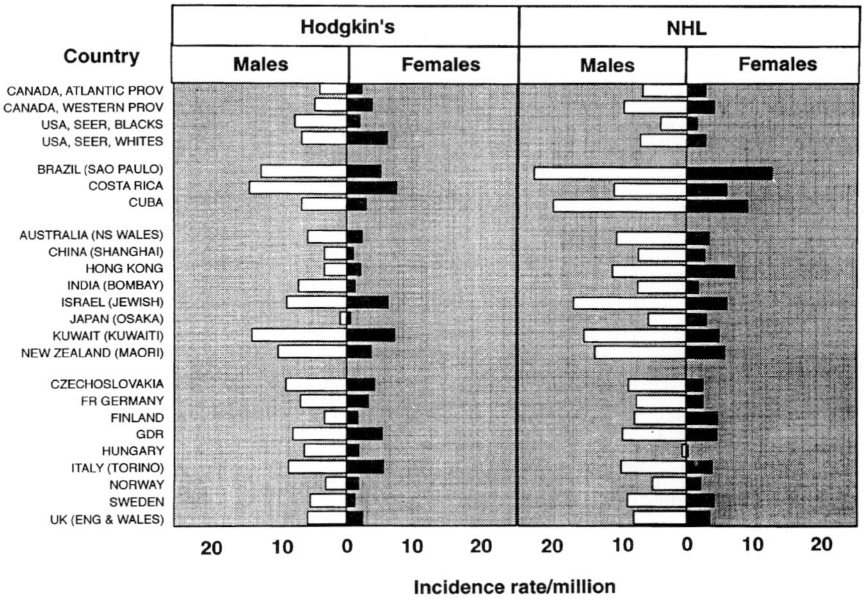

Figure 4. Annual incidence rates (per million population) in selected international sites for non-Hodgkin's lymphoma and Hodgkin's disease in children (adapted from Parkin et al, 1988).

that seen in other countries with an above-average incidence. The markedly higher incidence in regions of Africa is the result of endemic Burkitt lymphoma. Other areas reporting high rates of NHL include Brazil, Israel (Jewish), and Cuba. Intermediate rates occur in Australia and Costa Rica. The lowest rates are seen in Hungary, USA (among blacks), and Norway. The annual incidence rates in the USA are higher in whites compared with blacks, 9.1 and 5.4 per million population, respectively (Gurney et al, 1995). In most developed countries the incidence of NHL increases with age; however, in the USA this increase appears to be occurring primarily in males (Figure 5). The male predominance in the incidence of NHL is apparent throughout the world.

Aetiological considerations

Individuals with naturally occurring immunodeficiencies are at higher risk of developing NHL (Filipovich et al, 1992). In addition, the risk of NHL increases in populations with compromised immune status, such as organ transplant recipients (Penn, 1979) and HIV infection (Levine, 1993). Epstein–Barr virus-(EBV)-associated lymphomas are well-recognized among individuals with altered immune function (Young et al, 1989; Randhawa et al, 1992). The earlier observations by Burkitt in the distribution of endemic NHL in Africa lead to the discovery of EBV and the ongoing speculation on the role of EBV in the pathogenesis of African

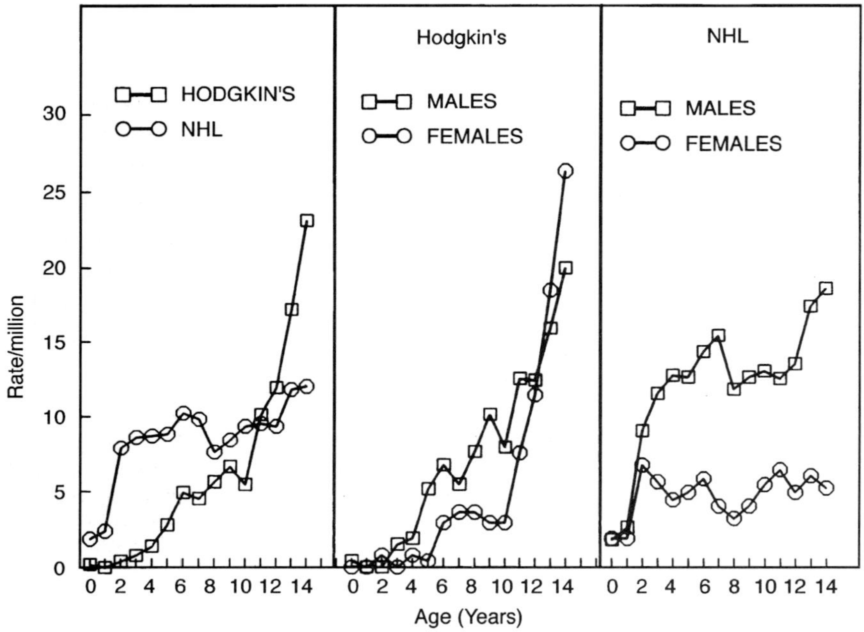

Figure 5. Age- and gender-specific annual incidence rates (per million population) for non-Hodgkin's lymphoma and Hodgkin's disease in children in the USA under the age of 15 years (adapted from Gurney et al, 1995).

Burkitt lymphoma. Burkitt lymphomas are characterized by one of three cytogenetic translocations, including t(8;14), t(8;22), and t(2;8). In each situation, the c-*myc* gene is juxtaposed to an immunoglobulin chain.

Studies of adult populations have provided evidence for an increased risk of NHL following exposure to pesticides and hair dyes (Blair et al, 1992), but no increase associated with exposure to radiation (Boice, 1992). The potential role of these or other environmental exposures in the aetiology of NHL in childhood is essentially unknown. Given the relatively low incidence of childhood NHL, the heterogeneity of the histologies with the diagnostic category of NHL and the potential importance of histologically-specific risk factors (as observed in adult NHL), it will be difficult to conduct large-scale epidemiological studies within the pediatric age group.

HODGKIN'S DISEASE

Incidence

In children, the occurrence of Hodgkin's disease is relatively rare and very infrequent before the age of 5 years (Figure 5). While there are international variations in the rates of Hodgkin's disease prior to the age of 15 (Figure 4), the annual incidence rate in most of the western developed countries is approximately 5–6 per million population (Parkin et al, 1988). The highest rates are reported from Brazil, Costa Rica and Kuwait, with the lowest rates seen in Japan, China (Shanghai), Hong Kong, Finland and Norway. There is a well established male predominance, as well as a higher incidence in whites compared to blacks (Gurney et al, 1995).

Hodgkin's disease is characterized by the striking bimodal age distribution, with the first peak occurring at approximately the age of 25, followed by a decline until approximately 40, at which point the incidence increases with increasing age. The bimodal pattern suggests that Hodgkin's disease represents two distinct aetiological processes, which is supported by the histological specificity seen within the two peaks.

Aetiological considerations

An infectious aetiology for Hodgkin's disease has for some time been a topic of interest. This interest resulted from reports of clusters of disease among individuals with possible personal contact (Grufferman and Delzell, 1984), as well as the unique epidemiological characteristics of the disease (Jarrett and Onions, 1992). The hypothesis that Hodgkin's disease in the young may be the result of a transmissible infectious agent has been supported by epidemiological studies of young adults. These studies demonstrated associations with childhood factors that would be likely to delay early exposure to infectious agents, including factors such as higher socio-economic status, fewer siblings in the family, living in a single-family home, and having fewer childhood playmates (Gutensohn and Cole, 1981). The demographic characteristics of Hodgkin's disease resemble those for the polio model.

For some time, EBV infection has been associated with Hodgkin's disease. Recent molecular biological studies of Hodgkin's disease tumour specimens have demonstrated the presence of EBV in some cases (Ambinder et al, 1993), increasing speculation of the potential importance of EBV in the pathogenesis of Hodgkin's disease.

As with childhood NHL, little is known about the aetiology of childhood Hodgkin's disease. The low incidence of Hodgkin's disease in the paediatric age group has limited the ability of investigators to conduct analytical epidemiological studies. Currently, a collaborative epidemiological study involving the two paediatric cooperative clinical trials groups is underway in the USA. This study will provide information on potential risk factors and biological characteristics in Hodgkin's cases under 15 years of age.

SUMMARY AND FUTURE AREAS OF INVESTIGATION

In contrast to the dramatic advances achieved in the treatment and characterization of leukaemia and lymphoma, relatively limited progress has been made in our understanding of the aetiology of these heterogeneous groups of cancers. With the realization that subgroups of cases can be characterized as biologically-distinct entities, the possibility that these heterogeneous groups of diseases may be aetiologically-distinct must be considered. If aetiological specificity exists for the biologically-defined subgroups, then the conduct of studies combining all cases would tend to obscure any subgroup-specific associations.

The suggestion that future studies need to have the ability to investigate risk factors within well-defined homogeneous subgroups poses several formidable obstacles. These include the ability systematically to classify cases into the relevant subgroups while having access to a sufficiently large population of cases. The latter is essential for allowing stratification of cases into biologically-distinct groups while maintaining acceptable statistical power to address hypotheses being tested.

The lack of information on the aetiology of childhood leukaemia may be changing in the near future. Presently, there are a number of large studies underway designed to address an array of hypotheses in childhood acute leukaemia. These studies, which include thousands of cases in North America and Europe, will be producing results during the next 2–3 years. The similarities in these studies will provide an opportunity to determine the consistency of findings within these diverse populations. Moreover, the potential exists for combined data analyses.

While there are several studies underway in childhood lymphomas, they are of a more limited scope because of the limited number of paediatric cases. Nonetheless, these studies should provide direction for future aetiological research relating to environmental and viral risk factors.

The use of established collaborative clinical trials groups for the conduct of epidemiological research has proven to be a useful and efficient approach (Robison et al, 1995). For our knowledge to advance in the aetiology of childhood leukaemias and lymphomas (as well as other paediatric cancers) multi-discipline and multi-institutional collaborations will be essential.

Acknowledgements

Support for this work was provided by the University of Minnesota Children's Cancer Research Fund and by National Cancer Institute grant T32 CA09607.

REFERENCES

Ambinder RF, Browning PJ, Lorenzana I et al (1993) Epstein–Barr virus and childhood Hodgkin's disease in Honduras and the United States. *Blood* **81:** 462–467.

Anderson RC (1955) Familial leukemia. *American Journal of Diseases of Childhood* **81:** 313–322.

Arico M, Comelli A, Bossi G et al (1993) Langerhans cell histiocytosis and acute leukemia: unusual association in two cases. *Medical Pediatric Oncology* **21:** 271–273.

Austin DF, Karp S, Dworsky R & Henderson BE (1975) Excess leukemia in cohorts of children born following influenza epidemics. *American Journal of Epidemiology* **101:** 77–83.

Bader JL & Miller RW (1978) Neurofibromatosis and childhood leukemia. *Journal of Pediatrics* **92:** 925–929.

Banks PM (1992) Changes in diagnosis of Non-Hodgkin's Lymphoma over time. *Cancer Research* **52:** 5453–5455.

Blair A, Linos A, Stewart PA et al (1992) Comments on occupational and environmental factors in the origin of Non-Hodgkin's lymphoma. *Cancer Research* **52:** 5501–5502.

Boice JD (1992) Radiation and Non-Hodgkin's lymphoma. *Cancer Research* **52:** 5489–5491.

Buckley JD, Robison LL, Swotinsky R et al (1989) Occupational exposures of parents of children with acute nonlymphocytic leukemia: a report from the Childrens Cancer Study Group. *Cancer Research* **49:** 4030–4037.

Buckley JD, Buckley CM, Ruccione K et al (1994) Epidemiological characteristics of childhood acute lymphocytic leukemia. Analysis by immunophenotype. *Leukemia* **8:** 856–864.

Bunin GR, Kuijten RR, Buckley JD et al (1993) Relation between maternal diet and subsequent primitive neuroectodermal brain tumors in young children. *New England Journal of Medicine* **329:** 536–541.

Cimino G, Lo Coco F, Biondi A et al (1993) ALL-1 gene at chromosome 11q23 is consistently altered in acute leukemia of early infancy. *Blood* **82:** 544–546.

Cotran RS, Kumar V & Robbins SL (eds) (1989) *Robbins Pathologic Basis of Disease*, 4th edn. Philadelphia, PA: WB Saunders Company.

Court-Brown WM & Doll R (1961) Leukemia in childhood and young adult life. *British Medical Journal* **1:** 981–988.

Creutzig U, Ritter J, Ludwig WD et al (1993) Classification of morphologic, immunologic and cytogenetic parameters- occurrence of subtypes in study AML-BFM-87. *Klinical Padiatrics* **205:** 272–280.

Crist W, Carroll A, Shuster J et al (1990) Philadelphia chromosome positive childhood acute lymphoblastic leukemia. Clinical and cytogenetic characteristics and treatment outcome. A Pediatric Oncology Group Study. *Blood* **76:** 489–494.

Doll R, Evans HJ & Darby SC (1994) Paternal exposure not to blame. *Nature* **367:** 678–680.

Eatough JP & Henshaw DL (1993) Radon and monocytic leukemia in England. *Journal of Epidemiology and Community Health* **47:** 506–507.

Ekelund H, Finnstrom O, Gunnarskog J et al (1993) Administration of vitamin K to newborn infants and childhood cancer. *British Medical Journal* **307:** 89–91.

Farwell J & Flannery JT (1984) Cancer in relatives of children with central nervous system tumors. *New England Journal of Medicine* **311:** 749–753.

Filipovich AH, Mathur A, Kamat D & Shapiro RS (1992) Primary immunodeficiences: genetic risk factors for lymphoma. *Cancer Research* **52:** 5465–5467.

Ford AM, Ridge SA, Cabrera ME et al (1993) *In utero* rearrangements in the trithorax related oncogene in infant leukemias. *Nature* **363:** 358–360.

Gardner MJ (1991) Father's occupational exposure to radiation and the raised level of childhood leukemia near the Sellafield Nuclear Plant. *Environmental Health Perspectives* **94:** 5–7.

German J, Bloom D & Passarge E (1979) Bloom's syndrome. VII. Progress report for 1978. *Clinical Genetics* **15:** 361–367.

Gibel W & Lohs K (1975) Carcinogenic, hematotoxic and hepatotoxic effects of organic phosphate pesticides. *Environmental Quality and Safety* **4:** 232–234.

Golding J, Greenwood R, Birmingham K & Mott M (1992) Childhood cancer, intramuscular vitamin K, and pethidine given during labor. *British Medical Journal* **305:** 341–346.

Greaves MF (1988) Speculations on the cause of childhood acute lymphoblastic leukemia. *Leukemia* **2:** 120–125.

Greaves MF, Colman SM, Beard MEJ et al (1993) Geographical distribution of acute lymphoblastic leukaemia subtypes: second report of the collaborative group study. *Leukemia* **7:** 27–34.

Grufferman S & Delzell E (1984) Epidemiology of Hodgkin's disease. *Epidemiologic Reviews* **6:** 76–106.

Gurney JG, Severson RK, Davis S & Robison LL (1995) Incidence of childhood cancer in the United States: gender-, race-, and 1-year age-specific rates by histology. *Cancer* **75:** 2186–2195.

Gutensohn NM & Cole P (1981) Childhood social environment and Hodgkin's disease. *New England Journal of Medicine* **304:** 135–140.

Hecht F & Hecht BK (1990) Cancer in ataxia-telangiectasia patients. *Cancer Genetics and Cytogenetics* **46:** 9–19.

Henderson ES & Lister TA (eds) (1990) *Leukemia*. Philadelphia: WB Saunders Company.

Jablon S, Tachikawa K & Belsky JL (1971) Cancer in Japanese exposed as children to atomic bombs. *Lancet* **i:** 927–931.

James WH (1990) Further evidence for the hypothesis that one cause of infant leukemia is infection. *Paediatric Perinatology and Epidemiology* **4:** 113–117.

Jarrett R & Onions D (1992) Viruses and Hodgkin's disease. *Leukemia* **6:** 14–17.

Kennedy MA, Gonzalez-Sarmiento R, Kees UR et al (1991) HOX11, a homeobox-containing T-cell oncogene on human chromosome 10q24. *Proceedings of the National Academy of Sciences of the USA* **88:** 8900–8904.

Kersey JH, Sabad A, Gajl-Peczalska K et al (1973) Acute lymphoblastic leukemia cells with T (thymus-derived) lymphocyte markers. *Science* **182:** 1355–1356.

Klebanoff MA, Read JS, Mills JL et al (1993) The risk of childhood cancer after neonatal exposure to vitamin K. *New England Journal of Medicine* **329:** 905–908.

LeBeau MM, Larson RA, Bitter MA et al (1983) Association of inversion of chromosome 16 with abnormal marrow eosinophils in acute myelomonocytic leukemia: a unique cytogenetic-clinicopathological association. *New England Journal of Medicine* **309:** 630–636.

LeBeau MM, Albain KS, Larson, RA et al (1986) Clinical and cytogenetic correlations in 63 patients with therapy-related myelodysplastic syndromes and acute non-lymphocytic leukemia: further evidence for characteristic abnormalities of chromosomes 5 and 7. *Journal of Clinical Oncology* **4:** 325–345.

Leisenring WM, Breslow NE, Evans IE et al (1994) Increased birth weights of National Wilms' Tumor Study patients suggest a growth factor excess. *Cancer Research* **54:** 4680–4683.

Levine AM (1993) AIDS-related malignancies: the emerging epidemic. *Journal of the National Cancer Institute* **85:** 1382–1397.

Linet MS (ed) (1985) *The Leukemias: Epidemiological Aspects.* New York: Oxford Press.

Maklin MT (1960) Inheritance of cancer of the stomach and large intestine in man. *Journal of the National Cancer Institute* **24:** 551–571.

McKinney PA, Cartwright RA, Saiu JMT et al (1987) The intra-regional epidemiological study of childhood cancer (IRESCC): a case–control study of aetiological factors in leukaemia and lymphoma. *Archives of Diseases of Childhood* **62:** 279–287.

McLaughlin JR, Clarke EA, Nishri ED & Anderson TW (1993) Childhood leukemia in the vicinity of Canadian nuclear facilities. *Cancer Causes and Control* **4:** 51–58.

Miller BA, Ries LAG, Hankey BF et al (1993) SEER Cancer Statistics Review: 1973–1990, National Cancer Institute. NIH Pub. No. 93–2789, p XXVII.5.

Olshan AF (1986) Wilms' tumor overgrowth and fetal growth factors: a hypothesis. *Cancer Genetics and Cytogenetics* **21:** 303–307.

Parkin DM, Stiller CA, Draper GJ et al (eds) (1988) International Incidence of Childhood Cancer, IARC Scientific Publications No. 87, Lyon, France.

Penn I (1979) Tumor incidence in human allograft recipients. *Transplant Proceedings* **11:** 1047–1051.

Peters JM, Preston-Martin S, London SJ et al (1994) Processed meats and risk of childhood leukemia (California, USA). *Cancer Epidemiology Biomarkers and Prevention* **5:** 195–202.

Pierce MI, Borges WH, Heyn R et al (1969) Epidemiological factors and survival experience in 1770 children with acute leukemia. *Cancer* **23:** 1296–1304.

Preston DL, Kusumi S, Tomonaga M et al (1994) Cancer incidence in atomic bomb survivors. Part III: Leukemia, lymphoma and multiple myeloma, 1950–1987. *Radiation Research* **137:** S68–S97.

Pui C-H, Ribeiro RC, Hancock ML et al (1991) Acute myeloid leukemia in children treated with epipodophyllotoxins for acute lymphoblastic leukemia. *New England Journal of Medicine* **325:** 1682–1687.

Ramot B & Magrath I (1982) Hypothesis: the environment is a major determinant of the immunological sub-type of lymphoma and acute lymphoblastic leukemia in children. *British Journal of Haematology* **50:** 183–189.

Randhawa PS, Jaffe R, Demetris AJ et al (1992) Expression of Epstein–Barr virus-encoded small RNA (by the EBER-1 gene) in liver specimens from transplant recipients with post-transplantation lymphoproliferative disease. *New England Journal of Medicine* **327:** 1710–1714.

Robison LL & Neglia JP (1987) Epidemiology of Down syndrome and childhood acute leukemia. In McCoy EE and Epstein CJ (eds) *Oncology and Immunology of Down Syndrome,* pp 19–32. New York: Alan Liss, Inc.

Robison LL, Buckley JD, Daigle AE et al (1989) Maternal drug use and risk of childhood nonlymphoblastic leukemia among offspring. An epidemiologic investigation implicating marijuana. (A report from the Childrens Cancer Study Group.) *Cancer* **63:** 1904–1911.

Robison LL, Buckley JD & Bunin G (1995) Assessment of environmental and genetic factors in the etiology of childhood cancers: the Childrens Cancer Group epidemiology program. *Environmental Health Prospectives* **103:** (in press).

Ross JA, Davies SM, Potter JD & Robison LL (1994) Epidemiology of childhood leukemia with a focus on infants. *Epidemiologic Reviews* **16:** 243–272.

Savitz DA, Wachtel H, Barnes FA et al (1988), Case–control study of childhood cancer and exposure to 60–Hz magnetic fields. *American Journal of Epidemiology* **128:** 21–38.

Secker-Walker LM, Berger R, Fernaux P et al (1992) Prognostic significance of the balanced t(1;9) and unbalanced der(19) t(1;19) translocations in acute lymphoblastic leukemia. *Leukemia* **6:** 363–369.

Severson RK, Buckley JD, Woods WG et al (1993) Cigarette smoking and alcohol consumption of parents of children with acute myeloid leukemia: an analysis within morphologic subgroups—a report from the Childrens Cancer Group. *Cancer Epidemiology Biomarkers and Prevention* **2:** 433–439.

Shaw MP, Eden Ob, Grace E et al (1992) Acute lymphoblastic leukemia and Klinefelter's syndrome. *Pediatric Hematolology and Oncology* **9:** 81–85.

Shu XO, Gao YT, Linet MS et al (1987) Chloramphenicol use and childhood leukaemia in Shanghai. *Lancet* **2:** 934–937.

Shu XO, Gao YT, Brinton LA et al (1988) A population-based case–control study of childhood leukemia in Shanghai. *Cancer* **62:** 635–644.

Shu XO, Reaman GH, Lampkin B et al (1994) Association of paternal diagnostic X-ray exposure with risk of infant leukemia. *Cancer Epidemiology Biomarkers and Prevention* **3:** 645–653.

Siegel M (1993) Smoking and leukemia: evaluation of a causal hypothesis. *American Journal of Epidemiology* **1:** 1–9.

Stevens RG (1993) Biologically based epidemiological studies of electric power and cancer. *Environmental Health Perspective* **101 (supplement 4):** 93–100.

Stewart A, Webb J & Hewitt D (1958) A survey of childhood malignancies. *British Medical Journal* **ii:** 1495–1507.

Stone RM & Mayer RJ (1990) The unique aspects of acute promyelocytic leukemia. *Journal of Clinical Oncology* **8:** 1913–1921.

Strong LC (1984) Genetics, etiology and epidemiology of childhood cancer. In Sutow, WW, Fernbach, DJ & Vietti, TJ (eds) *Clinical Pediatric Oncology*, 3rd edn. St Louis: CV Mosby.

Tu J & Li FP (1983) Incidence of childhood tumors in Shanghai, 1973–1977. *Journal of the National Cancer Institute* **70:** 589–592.

Van Duijn CM, van Steensel-Moll HA, Coebergh JW & van Zanen GE (1994) Risk factors for childhood acute non-lymphocytic leukemia: an association with maternal alcohol consumption during pregnancy? *Cancer Epidemiology Biomarkers and Prevention* **3:** 457–460.

Van-Steensel Moll HA, Valkenburg HA et al (1985) Are maternal fertility problems related to childhood leukaemia? *International Journal of Epidemiology* **14:** 555–559.

Vianna NJ, Kovasznay B, Polan A & Ju C (1984) Infant leukemia and paternal exposure to motor vehicle exhaust fumes. *Journal of Occupational Medicine* **26:** 679–682.

Viel JF (1993) Radon exposure and leukaemia in adulthood. *International Journal of Epidemiology* **22:** 627–631.

Volgelstein B, Civin CI, Preisinger AC et al (1990) RAS gene mutations in childhood acute myeloid leukemia: a Pediatric Oncology Group Study. *Genes, Chromosomes & Cancer* **2:** 159–162.

Wertheimer N & Leeper E (1979) Electrical wiring configurations and childhood cancer. *American Journal of Epidemiology* **109:** 273–284.

Woods WG, Roloff JS, Lukens JN et al (1981) The occurrence of leukemia in patients with Shwachman syndrome. *Journal of Pediatrics* **99:** 425–428.

Woods WG, Nesbit ME, Buckley J et al (1985) Correlation of chromosome abnormalities with patient characteristics, histologic subtype and induction success in children with acute non-lymphocytic leukemia. *Journal of Clinical Oncoloy* **3:** 3–11.

Yeazel MW, Buckley JD, Woods WG et al (1995) History of maternal fetal loss and increased risk of childhood acute leukemia at an early age. *Cancer* **75:** 1718–1727.

Young L, Alfieri C, Hennessy K et al (1989) Expression of Epstein–Barr virus transformation-associated genes in tissues of patients with EBV lymphoproliferative disease. *New England Journal of Medicine* **321:** 1080–1085.

Zipursky A, Peeters M & Poon A (1987) Megakaryoblastic leukemia and Down's syndrome—review. *Progress in Clinical and Biological Research* **246:** 33–56.

2

Some recent developments in the pathology of acute lymphoblastic leukaemias and non-Hodgkin lymphomas in children

RICHARD L. CARTER
KEITH P. McCARTHY

There have been major advances in our understanding of the pathology of paediatric lymphoid malignancies over the last decade, due mainly to developments in immunocytochemistry, cytogenetics and molecular biology. The subject has become large and increasingly complex and, in this account, we concentrate on two aspects: the acute lymphoblastic leukaemias and non-Hodgkin lymphomas.

GENERAL ASPECTS OF LABORATORY DIAGNOSIS

The laboratory diagnosis of malignant lymphoid proliferations in children is often difficult and draws on immunocytochemistry and, increasingly, cytogenetics and molecular biology. It is therefore essential that biopsies of bone marrow, lymph nodes and other tissues are carefully planned and that adequate amounts of material are collected in an appropriate form. Tissue may be required variously for cytological smears and imprints, cytocentrifuge concentrates, routine histopathology, immunocytochemistry, short-term culture, extraction of DNA and/or RNA, and sometimes for virology and other purposes. Biopsies need to be handled and processed with care: crushed and ill-fixed material may yield only a partial diagnosis, or no diagnosis at all, and the importance of consistent, high-quality morphology cannot be over-emphasized.

The laboratory diagnosis of leukaemia or lymphoma requires a clear initial *exclusion* of reactive lymphoid changes, which, in young children, can be extremely florid, and of the paediatric (non-lymphohaematopoietic) round-cell malignancies. Some presentations of disseminated alveolar rhabdomyosarcoma and neuroblastoma, for example, may simulate acute leukaemia or lymphoma.

Baillière's Clinical Paediatrics—
Vol. 3, No. 4, November 1995
ISBN 0–7020–2075–3

Table 1. Antibodies commonly used in the tissue diagnosis of lymphoblastic leukaemias and lymphomas.

	Chemistry	Distribution	Comments
CD1a	Part of a family of 5 genes: structure similar to MHC Class 1 molecules	Cortical thymocytes, dendritic cells	Expression is minorly related with TCR and MHC class 1 expression
CD2	Interacts with CD58 to form adhesion pair, through which signal translocation may occur	All mature T-cells, NK cells and thymocytes	
CD3	Actually a complex of five peptides—γ, δ, ε, ν and ξ—associated with the T-cell receptor, and involved with signal translocation	Increasing expression with T-cell maturation	Paraffin antibody available
CD4	Co-receptor with TCR for binding antigen in association with MHC class II	Most thymocytes (also CD8 +ve) and T-helper cells (CD8 –ve): monocytes and macrophages	HIV-binding receptor
CD5	T-cell activation and proliferation: CD5 +ve B-cells produce polyreactive antibodies	Most thymocytes, all mature T-cells and a subset of mature B-cells	Binds to CD72
CD7	Unknown	Primitive haematopoietic cells, thymocytes, many mature T-cells	
CD8	Co-receptor with TCR for binding antigen in association with MHC class I	Most thymocytes (also CD4 +ve) and CD4 –ve mature T-cells	
CD10	Neutral endopeptidase which clears various peptides including enkephalins and angiot?	Wide: early B and T cells, some myeloid cells, bone marrow stromal cells, some epithelia, some soft tissues and glia	
CD13	Aminopeptidase, possibly involved in peptide-mediated signalling	Myeloid precursors and mature myeloid cells including monocytes: also some epithelia and soft tissues	
CD15	Involved in cell adhesion and phagocytosis by myeloid cells	Mature myeloid cells including monocytes, adeno-carcinomas and Reed–Sternberg and Hodgkin cells	Binds to CD62 and ELAM-1: paraffin antibody available
CD19	Regulation of B-cell proliferation	Early B-cell precursors and mature B-cells (not plasma cells); follicular dendritic cells	Paraffin antibody available

CD20	Regulation of B-cell activation and proliferation:? a calcium channel	B-cell precursors and mature B-cells (not plasma cells)	
CD21	Regulation of B-cell activation and proliferation	Mature B cells: follicular dendritic cells; some thymocytes: some epithelia	EBV-receptor
CD22	Cell adhesion to monocytes, T-cells, B-cells and erythrocytes	B-cell precursor and some mature B-cells: hairy cell leukaemia	
CD25	IL-2 receptor comprises α and β subunits; binding with IL-2 reduces activation and proliferation	Activated T-cells, B-cells and monocytes	
CD30	Member of nerve growth factor receptor family: function uncertain	Activated T-cells and B-cells. Hodgkin and Reed–Sternberg cells: some cases of embryonal carcinoma	Paraffin antibody available
CD33	Function unknown	Myeloid precursors, monocytes	
CD34	Function unknown: high degree of potential N-linked and O-linked glycosylatin suggests possible role in cell adhesion	Primitive haematopoietic precursors: endothelium	
CD45	Four isoforms are relevant—CD45RA, RB, RC and RO—found by alternative splicing; function appears to be signal translocation	All haematopoietic cells (except erythroid cells)	Paraffin antibody available (detects all isoforms)
CD45RO	Splice variant of CD45	Memory T-helper cells (not naive T-cells)	Specific paraffin antibody available
CD68	Lysosomal glycoprotein of uncertain function	Monocytic cells, basophils, neutrophils and large lymphocytes: hepatocytes and renal epithelium	Paraffin antibody available
EMA	Found on secretory epithelia	Many epithelia, some soft tissues, large-cell anaplastic lymphoma	Paraffin antibody available
Tdt	Terminal deoxynucleotide transferase: inserts nucleotides randomly at junctions during antigen receptor gene re-arrangement	Early B-cell and T-cell precursors	

Notes. 'CD numbers' refer to 'cluster determination' which are statistically-derived groups of antibodies apparently reacting with epitopes on the same antigen. This has proved invaluable in clarifying the confusion in antibody terminology and in facilitating research into the characterization of cell-surface antigens.

Immunocytochemistry

Immunocytochemistry is an adjunct, rather than a supplement, to meticulous conventional morphology. A useful introduction to the principles of immunohistochemistry and to the other special investigations considered here, may be found in Section 30, 'Diagnostic and Investigative Techniques', in the *Oxford Textbook of Pathology* (see McGee et al, 1992). A wide range of techniques can be performed on cell suspensions and cytocentrifuge preparations, smears, imprints and cryostat or routinely-processed histological sections. Frozen sections offer the advantage of better preservation of more epitopes so that a wider range of diagnostic antibodies can be used. The disadvantages are the practical problems of initial collection and storage of material, the small amounts of tissue and the poor preservation of cytological detail. Immunocytochemistry in fixed, conventionally-processed biopsy tissues has greatly improved with the introduction of better demonstration systems (sometimes including predigestion of sections with proteolytic enzymes) and the wide use of monoclonal antibodies. Microwave heating of tissue sections will enhance staining of existing isotopes and also unmasks other epitopes which are not usually demonstrable in routine paraffin sections. Antibodies commonly used in the immunocytological diagnosis of leukaemias and lymphomas are listed in Table 1.

Cytogenetics

The traditional methods require suspensions of living cells which are capable of mitosis. If colchicine is added, they are arrested in metaphase when the chromosomes have replicated and separated. 'Metaphase spreads' are then obtained by lysing the cells and staining the chromosomes with various agents. Giemsa produces a pattern of G-bands or (after treatment with hot alkali) R-bands; quinacrine staining reveals q-bands. Whichever method is used, the staining patterns obtained are unique for each chromosome, and karyotypic abnormalities can be identified and localized. The precise molecular basis of banding remains unclear. More recently, molecular techniques such as fluorescent in situ hybridization (FISH) have been developed. These methods make use of fluorescence-labelled DNA probes which bind in a highly specific fashion to complementary sequences: they are therefore applicable to interphase (non-dividing) cells and can be used on fixed tissues. FISH techniques are useful for demonstrating structural chromosomal abnormalities in neoplastic lymphoid cells, particularly translocations, and for detecting small-volume residual disease.

Gene rearrangement studies

These studies derive from two principal techniques, restriction enzyme analysis (REA) and the polymerase chain reaction (PCR).

First described by Southern in 1975, *restriction enzyme analysis* employs various bacterial restriction endonucleases which cleave DNA into oligomeric sequences specific for each enzyme. Subsequent rearrangement of the DNA fragments will alter the relevant positions of the cleavage sites and so produce DNA segments of different lengths. These are separated by electrophoresis in an agarose gel and then transferred to a permanent medium such as nitrocellulose or nylon membrane—the part of the method which is actually 'Southern blotting'. In order to visualize the DNA fragments of interest, a complementary radiolabelled DNA probe is hybridized to the electrophoresed DNA at a stringency sufficiently high to prevent non-specific binding. A radiograph is then prepared from the blot. A band in a position different to that of the germ line band indicates DNA fragments of different mobility (and thus of different size) compared with germ line; if polymorphisms are excluded, this finding is diagnostic for gene rearrangement. The original radioactive probes are now largely superseded by biotinylated or fluorescence-labelled probes. The main disadvantages of REA are that the technique requires sizeable amounts of biopsy tissue and expensive equipment, and it is slow. The method will reveal gene rearrangements in 2–5 tumour cells/100 normal cells, a level of sensitivity which is acceptable for primary diagnosis but not for detecting and monitoring low-volume residual disease.

The fundamental principles of the *polymerase chain reaction* (PCR) have been described in many articles and books, including the *Oxford Textbook of Pathology* (McGee et al, 1992). Compared to REA, PCR requires little tissue (and can be applied to routinely-processed biopsies) and it is rapid and cheap. It is, however, capable of reliably amplifying sequences of at most a few kilobases—and the shorter the sequence the better. Although many genetic rearrangements appear to be constant at a cytogenetic level, the breakpoints may occur over many kilobases and are thus not amenable to direct amplification by PCR. It is the translocations which cluster at particular breakpoints which are best suited for PCR analysis. Certain translocations with variable breakpoints may, however, result in an expressed fusion gene and, in these circumstances, the corresponding mRNA can be amplified by reverse transcriptase PCR (Morgan et al, 1989). Rearrangement of antigen receptor genes in lymphoid cells is detectable by PCR; however, the extreme variability of gene segments which are brought together to form the transcribed gene means that the design of appropriate primers must rely either on conserved sequences within the segment or on the use of gene segments which are known to be preferentially arranged in particular diseases. Methods which rely on conserved sequences within the antigen receptor gene segments are available for IgH, Ig-κ, TCR-β and TCR-γ genes (McCarthy et al, 1990, 1991, 1992). They are simple and quick but relatively insensitive, with significant levels of false-negative results. These may be due to the presence of as yet unsequenced gene segments which show marked sequence divergence, and to somatic hypermutation (Deane et al, 1991). Reliance on the detection of rearranged antigen receptor genes which are already known to occur in a given lymphoid neoplasm is, by definition, a limiting factor on the number of cases which can be identified.

CLASSIFICATION OF ACUTE LYMPHOBLASTIC LEUKAEMIAS AND NON-HODGKIN LYMPHOMAS

Acute lymphoblastic leukaemias (ALL) are classified according to the French American British (FAB) system and by immunophenotype. The FAB system, based primarily on cytology and cytochemistry, separated ALL into the subgroups described in Table 2 (Bennett et al, 1976). The main disadvantages of the FAB scheme are that it does not predict clinical behaviour and response to treatment. Immunophenotypic classifications satisfy both these requirements and are now widely used. There are three main categories, separating acute lymphoblastic leukaemias into B-lineage, T-lineage and null-lineage groups. The B-lineage cases are subdivided further into common (c), pre-B and B types. Common-ALL is now regarded as an early pre-B form of the disease. The defining immunophenotypes of the various categories of ALL are summarized in Table 3. Correlation between the FAB and immunophenotypic classifications is poor. For example, cases designated as L3 are seen only in B-lineage ALL, but not all B-ALL can be classified as L3; 95% of T-lineage ALL can be characterized as L1, but so can 90% of pre-B and early pre-B cases.

Non-Hodgkin lymphomas in children are distinctive in several respects (Murphy, 1980; Kjeldsberg et al, 1983; Wilson et al, 1984, 1987; Kjeldsberg and Wilson, 1986; Hutchison et al, 1988; Murphy et al, 1989). They are predominantly extranodal with diffuse, high-grade morphology and high proliferation rates. A leukaemic phase is common in many patients with lymphoblastic lymphomas, blurring the somewhat arbitrary distinction between leukaemic and lymphomatous processes—see later. Their morphological phenotypes are, however, restricted such that about 90% of all paediatric non-Hodgkin lymphomas can be grouped into one of three major descriptive categories:

1 small-cell lymphoblastic lymphomas of B- or T-lineage, closely related to the corresponding forms of acute lymphoblastic leukaemia;
2 a heterogeneous group of small non-cleaved cell lymphomas with a more mature B-cell immunophenotype which includes the endemic and sporadic forms of Burkitt lymphoma and a controversial group of Burkitt-like lymphomas; in American literature, this second category is often designated as undifferentiated, Burkitt and non-Burkitt;
3 a diverse and poorly characterized group of diffuse large-cell lymphomas which includes large-cell anaplastic lymphomas.

Lymphomas in the first two categories occur predominantly in children. The large-cell lymphomas occur in both children and adults. Other types of non-Hodgkin lymphoma, more familiar in older patients, are occasionally encountered in children; they include follicular lymphomas (centroblastic, centroblastic/centrocytic), sclerosing mediastinal B-cell lymphoma and peripheral T-cell lymphomas. A small proportion of paediatric lymphomas can be designated only as unclassifiable—malignant lymphoma (NOS) with or without a defined cell lineage—because either the biopsy material

Table 2. FAB classification of acute lymphoblastic leukaemias.

	L1	L2	L3
Cell size	Predominantly small (1–2 × small lymphocyte)	Larger but variable (>2 × small lymphocyte)	Large and homogeneous (>2 × small lymphocyte)
Nuclear features			
Shape	Regular, occasionally cleaved	Irregular, often cleaved	Regular and rounded
Nucleoli	None or small	One or more, often large	Prominent, possibly vesicular
Chromatin	Either dispersed or clumped, but constant	Either dispersed or clumped and variable in a single case	Finely stippled
Cytoplasmic features			
Amount	Scanty	Scanty to moderate	Moderate
Basophilia	Slight	Variable, possibly deep	Deep
Vacuolation	Variable	Variable	Prominent

Table 3. Immunophenotypic classification of acute lymphoblastic leukaemias.

Early pre-B ALL	CD1a–	CD10+	CD19+	Tdt+	CIgμ–		
Pre-B ALL	CD1a+	CD10+	CD19+	Tdt+	CIgμ+		
B-ALL	CD1a+	CD10+/–	CD19+	Tdt–	Sigμ+		
T-ALL	CD1a+/–	CD2+	CD5+	CD7+	CD10–	CD19–	Tdt+
Early pre-B	CD1a+	CD2–	CD5–	CD7–	CD10–	CD19+/–	Tdt+

Notes. Tdt: terminal deoxynucleotide transferase; CIgμ: cytoplasmic immunoglobulin μ-chain expression, without surface localization; SIgμ: surface immunoglobulin μ-chain. All cases of early pre-B, pre-B and B-ALL are negative for CD2, CD5 and CD7.

is technically inadequate or the appearances fall outside conventionally recognized diagnostic categories.

Closer examination of each of the three main descriptive categories reveals a number of debatable conditions within them, and it is no surprise that incorporation of some forms of paediatric lymphomas into the large classification schemes devised for adults (National Cancer Institute, 1982; Stansfeld et al, 1988; Chan et al, 1994) remains controversial.

ACUTE LYMPHOBLASTIC LEUKAEMIAS

The operational distinction between acute lymphoblastic leukaemias and lymphoblastic lymphomas rests on the degree of bone marrow involvement, infiltration of 25% or more of the marrow population by lymphoblasts being designated as involvement by acute leukaemia.

Acute lymphoblastic leukaemia accounts for c. 80% of all paediatric leukaemias. Of the remainder, c. 15% are acute myeloid leukaemias and 5% are chronic myeloid leukaemias; chronic lymphocytic leukaemia in children is exceptionally rare. Leukaemia in infants often has characteristic clinical, immunophenotypic and chromosomal features (Katz et al, 1988).

c-ALL (early pre-B) is the commonest form of acute lymphoblastic leukaemia and is responsible for c. 65% of childhood cases, pre-B ALL for c. 20%, B-ALL for c. 4% and T-ALL for c. 12%. The remainder consists of null variants with no discernible lineage. The peak incidence for c-ALL is in children aged between 2 and 5 years, an observation which suggests that events in utero may contribute to pathogenesis: identical mutations of the MLL gene have been found in identical twins with c-ALL (Ford et al, 1993).

The distinctive epidemiological and demographic features of c-ALL (see Chapter 1) have attracted speculation that this form of acute lymphoblastic leukaemia may be associated with delayed exposure to some non-specific infective agent which stresses the immune system of small children at a relatively later time. If a previous leukaemogenic event has already caused a low-grade, subclinical lymphoid proliferation, this additional stress would be acting on a relatively larger population of atypical lymphoid cells and the probability of more genomic damage sustained during mitosis would be increased (Greaves and Alexander, 1993).

Immunocytochemistry

The clinical importance of establishing the various immunophenotypes that comprise acute lymphoblastic leukaemia has already been noted (Greaves et al, 1985). Common or early pre-B ALL is a favourable prognostic subgroup at all ages. Pre-B ALL has a higher risk of CNS involvement and bone marrow relapse, although there is no good evidence of a worse prognosis than in early pre-B cases. The t(1;19)(q23;q13) chromosomal abnormality is present in a proportion of patients. B-ALL, as distinct from marrow infiltration by Burkitt/Burkitt-like lymphoma, is uncommon and tends to occur in older patients. It has the same chromosomal translocations as Burkitt lymphoma (see later), although there are subtle cytological features that distinguish it. T-ALL frequently presents with mediastinal disease, and invasion of the CNS is common. Prognosis is traditionally regarded as poor but is improved by intensive chemotherapy; the T-cell immunophenotype itself is not an independent prognostic variable (Greaves et al, 1981). Two other categories need to be noted. As many as 20% of cases of childhood ALL co-express myeloid antigens, principally CD13 and 33 (Norton et al, 1987). These biphenotypic leukaemias may have a poor prognosis, particularly if an 11q23 rearrangement is also present (Raimondi et al, 1989; Pui et al, 1991). The other category is acute undifferentiated leukaemia, expressing neither lymphoid nor myeloid antigens. This group is reduced if additional molecular investigations are undertaken to demonstrate antigen receptor gene rearrangements; however, it should be borne in mind that such rearrangements occur in c. 20% of cases of otherwise typical acute myeloid leukaemia (Rovigatti et al, 1984).

Cytogenetics

Cytogenetic abnormalities can now be detected in 90–95% of patients with ALL (Pui et al, 1990b) albeit with varying frequencies in the different subgroups. Numerical abnormalities are more common than structural abnormalities, the latter occurring in c. 40% of cases (Pui et al, 1990). Only 5% of patients with ALL have 46 structurally normal chromosomes (Pui et al, 1990).

Numerical abnormalities. An almost complete continuum of chromosome numbers has been reported in ALL. The commonest structural abnormality is *hyperploidy*, occurring in 42% of patients with chromosome numbers ranging from 47 to 65 (Secker-Walker et al, 1989). These hyperdiploid cases have been subdivided into two groups, those with 47–50 chromosomes and those with 50 or more. The first group has no obvious clinical, morphological or prognostic features. The second group, by contrast, has a good prognosis. Many of these patients are aged between 2 and 5 years of age, and their leukaemic cells show an early pre-B immunophenotype. *Hypodiploidy* has been found in about 7% of patients. Chromosome numbers vary between 30 and 45, but the commonest abnormality is loss of a single chromosome, usually involving chromosome 20 (Pui et al, 1987). Rare cases have been reported with 66–73 chromosomes (*near diploidy*) or 82–94 chromosomes (*near tetraploidy*) (Pui et al, 1990). The blasts from such patients typically show extremely coarse chromatin. Near-tetraploid cases have a poor prognosis, and usually present at an older age with a T-immunophenotype (Pui et al, 1990). Approximately 10% of leukaemias have no demonstrable numerical or structural abnormalities in their chromosomes, but defects are almost certainly present which elude the current methods of cytogenetic analysis. The leukaemic blasts from many of these patients show a T-immunophenotype (Pui et al, 1990).

Numerical and structural karyotypic abnormalities are not mutually exclusive. *Pseudoploidy* (46 chromosomes with structural abnormalities) forms the largest single ploidy group—42%—and is associated with several unfavourable prognostic features: older age group and high total white blood cell counts at presentation, and immunophenotypes *other than* early pre-B (Secker-Walker et al, 1989).

Structural abnormalities. Although there is no single structural abnormality which is consistently associated with ALL, there are several chromosomal changes of diagnostic and prognostic importance which occur with moderate frequency. The Philadelphia chromsome (Ph^1), for example, is found in patients with c-ALL at frequencies of c. 25% in adults and c. 5% in children (Rowley, 1990). It is postulated that some examples of Ph^1 +ve c-ALL may have arisen as a result of blast crisis from a pre-existing subclinical or short-phase CML, an explanation which is consistent with the relative frequency of Ph^1 in adult and paediatric c-ALL. Whatever its origin, the detection of Ph^1 in c-ALL indicates an extremely poor prognosis (Fletcher et al, 1991). It is an independent variable, but is associated with older age and high white blood cell counts at presentation, and with CNS infiltration. The Ph^1 chromosome represents a balanced translocation involving the long arms of chromosomes 9 and 22—t(9;22)(p34;q12)—with the breakpoints occurring in the *bcr* and *abl* proto-oncogenes. The normal function of *bcr* is unknown, but *abl* is a tyrosine kinase which is involved in normal cell proliferation. The translocation results in an abnormal fusion gene (*bcr-abl*) which is transcribed and expressed. The gene product has increased tyrosine kinase activity and is thought to be implicated in leukaemogenesis (Lugo et al, 1990).

The translocation t(1;19)(p23;q13) is present in about 25% of pre-B-ALL and is an adverse prognostic factor. Many of these patients are non-white, present at an older age with high white blood cell counts, and lack hyperdiploidy (Shikano et al, 1986; Raimondi et al, 1990). This translocation involves a homeobox-containing gene (PBX-1) on chromosome 1 and a helix–loop–helix gene (E2A) on chromosome 19 (Kamps et al, 1990). The resulting fusion gene is transcribed and expressed. The two translocated genes are DNA-binding domains found in some transcriptional regulators, often those involved in development. The relevance of this translocation to the leukaemic process is unknown.

By conventional cytogenetics, c. 4% of T-ALL cases have either a deletion of chromsome 1 (del 1p) or a reciprocal translocation t(1;14), also involving this locus (Bernard et al, 1991). Analysis by PCR, however, indicates that the 1p deletion is present in as many as 25% of cases (Brown et al, 1990). The breakpoint (coincidentally called the Tal-deletion) is, in fact, upstream of Tal-1 and brings the Tal-1 gene under the influence of the SCR-5 gene enhancer (Breit et al, 1993). The 1p deletion is thought to be due to erroneous DNA excision by the recombinase system, a poorly characterized group of enzymes responsible for rearrangement of antigen receptor genes.

Rearrangements of 11q23 are found in a subgroup of patients who have a poor prognosis, often with high presenting white blood cell counts, co-expression of myeloid antigens (CD15) and presenting as infants aged less than 1 year (Pui et al, 1991). The translocation may involve a variety of other chromosomes including 4q21, 9p21 and 19p13 (Potter et al, 1993). The gene at 11q23 has recently been cloned and found to be a homeobox-containing gene named MLL (Ziemin-van der Poel et al, 1991).

Gene rearrangements

The immunoglobulin heavy-chain gene is rearranged early in B-lymphocyte ontogeny and is demonstrable in nearly all cases of early pre-B, pre-B and B-ALL, as detected by restriction enzyme analysis. The appreciable false-negative rate with PCR-based methods was noted earlier. T-ALL may show rearrangement of either TCR-β, TCR-γ or both genes. Rearrangement of the TCR-γ gene takes place early in T lymphocyte development; it may even occur in cells which will eventually bear only an α/β T cell receptor, thus explaining the occurrence of both β and γ rearrangements. A small percentage of T-ALL are of γ/δ lineage and have rearrangements of TCR-γ or -δ but not TCR-α or -β.

It is important to note that rearrangements of antigen receptor genes cannot be used as absolute indicators of cell lineage. Thus, heavy-chain gene rearrangements may occur in immunophenotypic T-ALL, and TCR-β or -γ genes may be arranged in the various immunophenotypically defined forms of B-ALL. This phenomenon is more likely to occur with IgH and TCR-γ genes than with Ig light-chain genes or the TCR-β gene. The incidence of cross-lineage, or promiscuous gene rearrangement in ALL approaches 25 to 30% (Kitchingman et al, 1985). Lineage infidelity of a similar order is also encountered in high-grade non-Hodgkin lymphomas (Davey et al, 1986).

Detection of minimal residual disease

Demonstration of minute amounts of residual leukaemia requires methods with a sensitivity of at least 1 in 10^4—i.e. 1 leukaemic cell/10 000 non-leukaemic cells (Potter et al, 1993). More sensitive methods with detection rates of c. 1 in 10^7 are at a high risk of contamination giving false-positive results. PCR-based techniques are widely used, monitoring either rearrangements of antigen receptor genes or abnormal chromosomes (Potter et al, 1993).

Antigen receptor genes offer an initially attractive target, but there are a number of disadvantages. The amplification process may fail because the primers are not homologous with the rearranged segments. The probes need to be specific for each patient since different leukaemic populations have different rearrangements and different N-regions. Thirdly, there is the problem of oligoclonality and clonal evolution. Approximately 40% of B-lineage ALL have multiple IgH rearrangements due to secondary rearrangements occurring in cells in which TdT is still active (Beishuizen et al, 1991). Chromosomal alterations such as t(9;22) t(1;19) and the Tal-1 deletion avoid the problems of secondary gene rearrangement but, once again, they suffer from the disadvantage of not being consistent features for any one form of ALL.

LYMPHOBLASTIC LYMPHOMA

Children with *B-lymphoblastic lymphoma* usually present with involvement of supradiaphragmatic lymph nodes and extranodal sites such as skin and occasionally bone. Dissemination to bone marrow, testes, ovaries and central nervous system is frequent. T-lymphoblastic lymphomas occur mainly in the mediastinum, often with pleural effusions and in peripheral lymph nodes. Spread to bone marrow is common. Involvement of intra-abdominal nodal groups by lymphoblastic lymphomas is rare. Morphological appearances are reasonably consistent (Nathwani et al, 1981; Kjeldsberg et al, 1983; Kjeldsberg and Wilson, 1986; Griffith et al, 1987; Chan et al, 1994) (Figure 1). No distinction can be drawn between

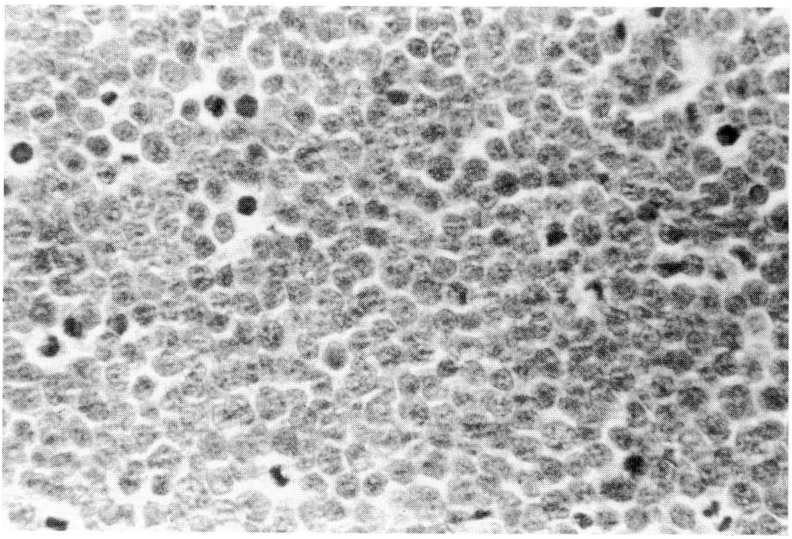

Figure 1. Lymphoblastic lymphoma, cervical lymph node.

lymphoblastic lymphomas of different lineage, nor between lymphoblastic lymphomas and acute lymphoblastic leukaemias. The malignant cells, arranged in diffuse sheets, are slightly larger than a mature small lymphocyte. Cellular and nuclear pleomorphism is slight. The nuclei are rounded or convoluted, with fine chromatin and inconspicuous nucleoli. Cytoplasm is scanty and weakly basophilic. Mitotic figures are abundant. The 'starry sky' appearance, due to apoptotic lymphoma cells and accumulations of phagocytic histiocytes, is variable: if present, it is more often focal than diffuse. Necrosis is sometimes extensive and may, in extreme examples, preclude a tissue diagnosis. Convoluted nuclei (Nathwani et al, 1981) are not a reliable distinguishing feature for T-lineage neoplasms. In a minority of cases, the lymphoblasts appear larger and more pleomorphic, such that the distinction from Burkitt and Burkitt-like lymphomas is difficult. The fine nuclear chromatin typical of lymphoblasts is, however, usually retained.

BURKITT LYMPHOMA; BURKITT-LIKE (syn. NON-BURKITT) LYMPHOMA

The endemic and sporadic forms of Burkitt lymphoma show a predominantly extranodal distribution of disease with predilection for the jaws, ileocaecal region, kidney, breasts and gonads: jaw tumours predominate in the endemic African form of the disease while ileocaecal masses predominate in sporadic cases. Mesenteric nodes may be involved but other forms of nodal disease, and marrow involvement, are uncommon. The morphological features of sporadic and endemic Burkitt lymphoma are indistinguishable (Kjeldsberg et al, 1983; Kjeldsberg and Wilson, 1986; Chan et al, 1994) (Figure 2). The malignant cells are slightly larger than lymphoblasts, and a little more pleomorphic. Rounded nuclei contain prominent (usually two to five) nucleoli and coarse chromatin. The cytoplasm is more abundant than in lymphoblasts, more basophilic and frequently contains lipid droplets which are best seen in smears and imprints. Mitotic figures are very numerous, and there is extensive tumour cell apoptosis with accumulation of phagocytic macrophages: the resulting 'starry sky' appearance is intense and usually seen throughout the sections. Necrosis is sometimes pronounced. The growth pattern is diffuse but a focal follicular arrangement is occasionally apparent, suggesting either an origin for Burkitt cells from follicular centre elements and/or a 'homing' migration of Burkitt cells to follicular regions (Mann et al, 1976).

The typical immunophenotype of Burkitt lymphoma is as follows: CD45+, CD10+, CD19+, CD20+, CD22+, SIgM+, T markers –, Tdt–.

Most cases have translocations of the c-*myc* proto-oncogene from chromosome 8 either into the Ig heavy chain locus on chromosome 14—t(8;14)—or, less commonly, to the Ig κ or λ light chain loci on chromosomes 2 or 22—t(2;8), t(8;22) (Nowell and Croce, 1990). The resulting deregulation of c-*myc* expression seems to be a critical event in the pathogenesis of Burkitt lymphoma (Magrath, 1990). The normal c-*myc* gene

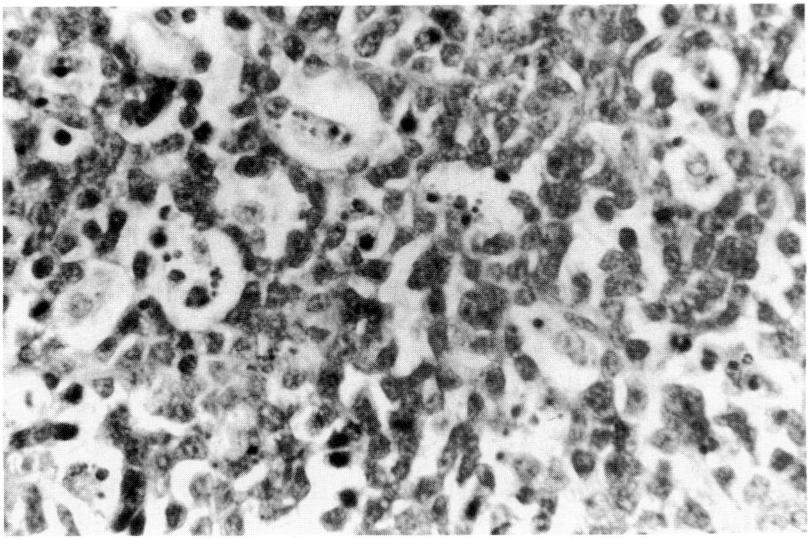

Figure 2. Endemic Burkitt's lymphoma: parotid mass.

product appears to be important in controlling cell division and differentiation, and tumours with translocated c-*myc* characteristically show extremely high rates of cell proliferation. EB viral genomes are regularly demonstrable in lymphoma cells from endemic cases but are only infrequently present in sporadic cases.

The morphological distinction between endemic and sporadic Burkitt lymphoma and the entity or entities variously known as *Burkitt-like* or *non-Burkitt lymphoma* remains controversial (Grogan et al, 1982; Miliauskas et al, 1982; Kjeldsberg et al, 1983; Kjeldsberg and Wilson, 1986; Kelly et al, 1987; Wilson et al, 1987; Hutchison et al, 1989; Chan et al, 1994). It has been described as 'often subtle, largely subjective, and a major source of disagreement in the pathology review process' (Kjeldsberg and Wilson, 1986)—Figure 3. Compared to endemic or sporadic Burkitt lymphoma, the cells are larger with more pleomorphic nuclei and fewer, but more prominent, nucleoli. 'Starry sky' appearances are variable. Mitotic figures are abundant. Certain distinction between Burkitt-like lymphomas, the uncommon pleomorphic variant of B-lymphoblastic lymphoma (see earlier), and B-lineage large cell lymphomas is sometimes impossible. The diagnosis in individual cases may be resolved by immunocytochemistry and/or cytogenetics. Recent molecular studies (Yano et al, 1992) comparing Burkitt and Burkitt-like lymphomas have not clarified these issues. A series of 18 Burkitt lymphomas showed consistent rearrangements of c-*myc*, *bcl-2* and *bcl-1*. The findings in 11 patients with Burkitt-like lymphomas (only one of whom was a child) revealed *bcl-2* rearrangements in three cases, no rearrangements of c-*myc* and no other abnormalities.

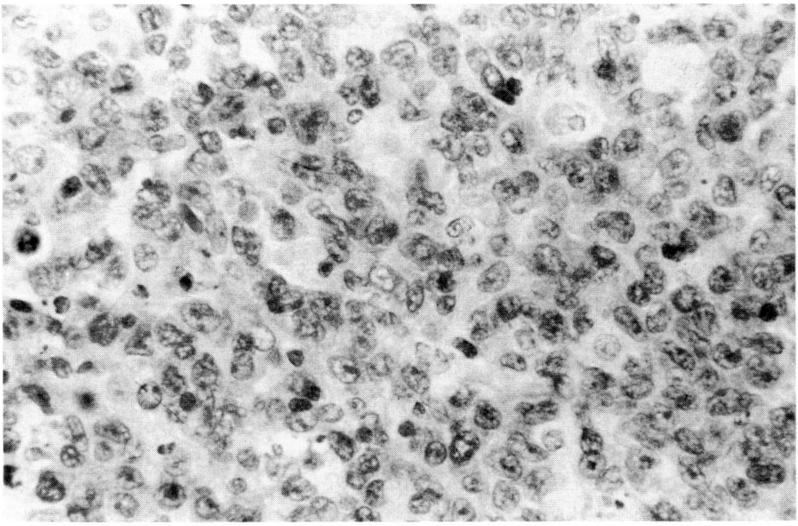

Figure 3. Burkitt-like lymphoma: ileocaecal mass.

The clinical implications of separating the Burkitt and Burkitt-like categories are predictably unclear. Some investigators claim that the distinction has prognostic implications in terms of response to treatment or median or overall survival, while others dispute any such association. It is worth noting that some studies included adults, treatment protocols changed during the sometimes long periods of time over which cases were collected, and many of the techniques now used in laboratory diagnosis were not available.

LARGE CELL LYMPHOMAS

This group of lymphomas is equally diverse in clinical presentation and in morphology. A wide variety of nodal and extranodal sites may be involved including peripheral and deep lymph nodes, skin, bones, gastrointestinal tract and lungs. Infiltration of CNS and bone marrow is uncommon. Most of the retrospective accounts of the pathology of paediatric large-cell lymphomas (Kjeldsberg et al, 1983; Kjeldsberg and Wilson, 1986; Nathwani et al, 1987; Hutchison et al, 1991) are based solely on microscopic morphology which served to distinguish two major categories: immunoblastic and large follicular centre cell. Each was subdivided further: immunoblastic lymphomas, for example, being separated into plasmacytoid, clear-cell and polymorphous forms. A proportion of cases remains unclassifiable. Many of the criteria used are drawn from the large classification schemes devised for adult patients (see earlier). The classification of paediatric large cell lymphomas has, however, changed within the last decade with the recognition of a new entity called *large-cell anaplastic, or Kil +, lymphoma.*

In 1982, Schwab and co-workers raised a monoclonal antibody against a Hodgkin disease cell line which reacted with Reed–Sternberg cells and also with scattered parafollicular lymphoid cells in normal reactive lymph nodes and tonsils. The antigen was designated Ki1 and was later codified in the CD system as CD30 (see Table 1). Expression of this Hodgkin disease-associated Ki1 antigen was then demonstrated immunocytochemically in about 5 to 10% of adult high-grade non-Hodgkin lymphomas of either T- or B-lineage, usually confined to a minority of the malignant cells, and—much more consistently—in an unusual large-cell lymphoma with distinctive growth pattern and cytological features which occurred in both children and adults (Stein et al, 1985). The tumour characteristically involved the sinus system of lymph nodes, showed intense cellular pleomorphism and for several years had been known as malignant histiocytosis. More examples were described, many of them in young people, and the clinical and pathological features of large-cell anaplastic lymphoma began to emerge (Kadin et al, 1986; O'Connor et al, 1987; Schnitzer et al, 1988; Delsol et al, 1988; Chan et al, 1989; Chott et al, 1990; Greer et al, 1991; Vecchi et al, 1993). The condition is now included in the updated Kiel classification (Stansfeld et al, 1988) and in the recent proposals for classification of lymphoid neoplasms by the International Lymphoma Study Group (Chan et al, 1994).

The clinical features are diverse and essentially the same as those listed for the general category of paediatric large-cell lymphomas. Involvement of skin or bone with nodal disease is particularly characteristic. The morphology is distinctive—Figure 4. In lymph nodes, the lymphomatous process is initially concentrated in the paracortical regions and sinuses, with preservation of follicles. The malignant cells are cohesive, larger and often intensely pleomorphic, including binucleate and multinucleate forms closely resembling Reed–Sternberg elements. They sometimes show evidence of phagocytosis. Nodular or diffuse fibrosis may occur. There is a variable accompanying infiltrate of eosinophils, plasma cells and histiocytes. Some groups have attempted to subclassify the atypical cells (Chan et al, 1989; Chott et al, 1990). Variant forms of large-cell anaplastic lymphoma have been described, including an apparently unique example with sarcomatoid features (Chan et al, 1990), cases with a high content of reactive histiocytes (Pileri et al, 1990) and the rather confusingly named small-cell variant (Kinney et al, 1993) in which the large anaplastic elements are inconspicuous and may become obvious only in subsequent relapsed disease.

The recognition that large-cell anaplastic lymphomas were lymphoid rather than histiocytic malignancies was based on immunophenotyping and the results of gene rearrangement studies. Immunocytochemical profiles are complex and, as in other lymphomas, may vary according to the use of frozen sections or paraffin wax sections. The typical immunophenotype is CD45+ or –, CD30+, EMA usually+. T-lineage cases will show CD3+, CD45RO+. The rare B-lineage cases will mark with pan B markers such as

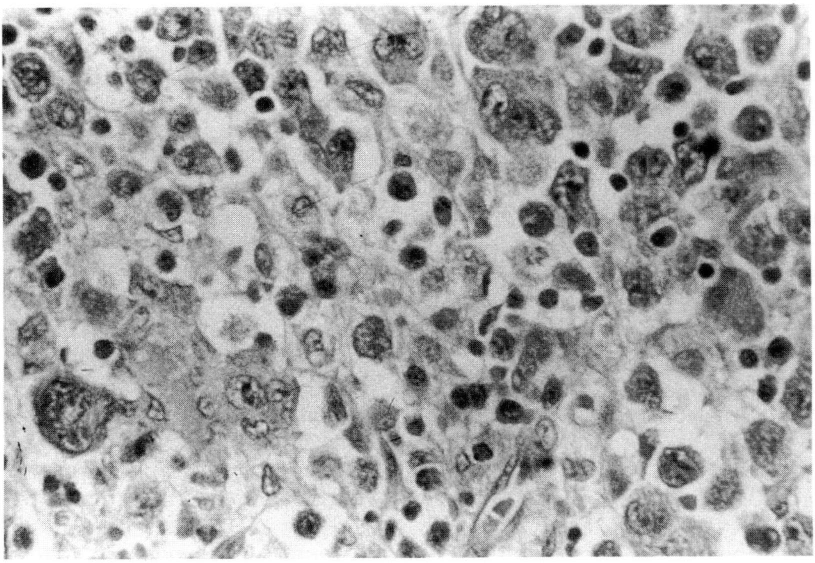

Figure 4. Large-cell anaplastic lymphoma: lytic bone lesion.

CD20. Null-lineage or indeterminate examples fail to react with B- or T-cell markers. Genotypic investigations (Stein et al, 1985; O'Connor et al, 1987; Schnitzer et al, 1988; Herbst et al, 1989) show a similar diversity. Gene rearrangements are reported in about two-thirds of cases. Rearrangement of T-cell receptor genes (TCR-β, -γ or both) are much more common than rearranged IgH genes. There is, however, an apparent discrepancy between the results of some of the gene rearrangement studies and the immunophenotypes which is at the moment unexplained. The lack of gene rearrangement in about one-third of cases is puzzling.

Cytogenetic changes also occur in large cell anaplastic lymphoma. A translocation t(2;5)(p23;q35) was originally described as characteristic of malignant histiocytosis by Morgan et al (1986), but several later investigators showed that this translocation was a feature of the newly recognized CD30+ large-cell anaplastic lymphoma (Kaneko et al, 1989; Rimokh et al, 1989; Le Beau et al, 1989; Bitter et al, 1990; Mason et al, 1990). The t(2;5) translocation does not involve breakpoints near the sites of the proto-oncogenes N-*myc* on chromosome 2 or c-*fms* on chromsome 5 (Morgan et al, 1989), but recent work indicates that the translocation may result in a fusion product of the nucleolar phosphoprotein gene (*npm*) on chromsome 5 and a protein tyrosine kinase gene (ALK) on chromosome 2. The resulting hybrid protein has tyrosine kinase activity (Pébasque et al, 1993; Morris et al, 1994; Orscheschek et al, 1995). The situation is analogous to the t(9;22)(q34;q12)—the Ph[1] chromosome—where the transcribed fusion gene product, *bcr-abl*, also has tyrosine kinase activity which may have implications for pathogenesis.

Although large-cell anaplastic lymphoma probably subsumes many examples of large-cell lymphomas in children (Hutchison et al, 1991), its status is still debatable in several respects. The pronounced morphological variability has already been noted. Immunocytochemical staining for CD30 is generally regarded as a diagnostic requirement, but the antibody can be capricious, and CD30 + lymphoid cells regularly occur in other high-grade, non-Hodgkin lymphomas of T- or B-lineage in adults (Stein et al, 1985; Piris et al, 1990) and even in some low grade follicular lymphomas (Piris et al, 1991). Staining in such cases is usually focal, in contrast to the diffuse and sometimes intense staining found in large cell anaplastic lymphomas, but not always. CD30 staining may occasionally occur in histiocytes and it has been described in some germ cell neoplasms: problems of false-positive and false-negative staining with this antibody are therefore extremely important (Pallesen, 1990).

The relationship between large-cell anaplastic lymphoma and other lymphomas is also problematic. In adults, the condition sometimes appears to evolve from mycosis fungoides, peripheral T cell lymphomas and, in particular, Hodgkin's disease. These two entities may be difficult or impossible to distinguish, and may indeed form part of a continuous spectrum (Leoncini et al, 1990). A distinction between them cannot be made on immunocytochemical grounds, and the t(2;5) translocation may perhaps occur in adults with Hodgkin's disease (Orscheschek et al, 1995). For the moment, large-cell anaplastic lymphoma can be regarded as a distinct clinicopathological entity although its definition may need to be modified in the light of new information.

Large-cell lymphomas which are CD30 *negative* represent a mixed group of rarities comprising B-lineage large-cell lymphoma of follicular origin (see next section), some of the peripheral T-cell lymphomas, and lymphomas of uncertain lineage and/or unclassifiable morphology. The sclerosing B-cell lymphomas of the mediastinum can also be included.

Published accounts of *peripheral T-cell lymphomas* in children have included the CD30+ large-cell anaplastic lymphomas of T-lineage (Leake et al, 1989; Lee et al, 1991; Gordon et al, 1993). The small numbers of CD30 *negative* cases are predictably varied and are composed of pleomorphic large cells, mixed large and medium cells, immunoblast-like cells, and one example of a low-grade angioimmunoblastic type. EBV DNA was present in four of six examples described from Taiwan; HTLV-1 proviral genome was not demonstrated (Lee et al, 1991).

Sclerosing B-cell lymphomas of the mediastinum occur mainly in adolescents and young adult females, presenting as discomfort in the chest, dyspnoea and other symptoms referable to superior caval obstruction. They show a diffuse arrangement, composed of large cleaved and non-cleaved follicular centre cells set in fibrous tissue which may assume various patterns: a fine interstitial arrangement, formation of more discrete compartments or broad bands (Perrone et al, 1986; Lamarre et al, 1989; Carr et al, 1993). Tissue diagnosis is frequently difficult: biopsies are often small and crushed (partly because of the fibrosis), necrosis is common, and the epithelioid appearances of the lymphoma cells may lead to confusion with Hodgkin's disease, thymoma or even seminoma. Immunophenotyping confirms B-lineage, and rearrangement of IgH and L genes has been described in a few cases (Lamarre et al, 1989). These lymphomas probably arise from the normal B cell population present in the thymic medulla (Isaacson et al, 1987).

FOLLICULAR LYMPHOMAS

Low- and intermediate-grade B-lineage follicular lymphomas are very rare in children, contributing only 0–3% in most large series (Frizzera and Murphy, 1979; Winberg et al, 1981; Ribeiro et al, 1992). The paediatric cases differ from the relatively common follicular lymphomas in adults in several respects. Disease is usually localized to lymph nodes and/or tonsils, without bone marrow involvement, and B symptoms are rare. Mixed follicular and diffuse forms are more common than the pure follicular form, and most paediatric cases are composed of large cells or mixtures of large cells and small cells. The tissue diagnosis is straightforward provided that it is always realized that lymphadenopathy with florid reactive changes is very common in children while follicular lymphomas are very rare. The cure rate for low-stage follicular lymphoma in children is excellent.

REFERENCES

Beishuizen A, Hahlen K, Hagemeijer A et al (1991) Multiple rearranged immunoglobulin genes in childhood acute lymphoblastic leukemia of precursor B-cell origin. *Leukemia* **5:** 657–667.

Bennett JM, Catovsky D, Daniel M-T et al (1976) Proposals for the classification of the acute leukaemias. *British Journal of Haematology* **33:** 451–458.

Bernard J, Lecointe N, Jonveaux P et al (1991) Two site-specific deletions and t(1; 14) translocation restricted to human T-cell acute leukaemias disrupt the 5′ part of the tal-1 gene. *Oncogene* **6:** 1477–1488.

Bitter MA, Franklin WA, Larson RA et al (1990) Morphology in Ki-1 (CD30)-positive non-Hodgkin's lymphoma is correlated with clinical features and the presence of a unique chromosomal abnormality, t(2;5)(p23;q35). *American Journal of Surgical Pathology* **14:** 305–316.

Breit TM, Beishuizen A, Ludwig W-D et al (1993) tal-1 deletions in T-cell acute lymphoblastic leukemia as PCR target for detection of minimal residual disease. *Leukemia* **7:** 2004–2011.

Brown L, Cheng J-T, Chen Q et al (1990) Site-specific recombination of the tal-1 gene is a common occurrence in human T cell leukemia. *EMBO Journal* **9:** 3343–3351.

Carr TF, Lockwood L, Stevens RF et al (1993) Childhood B cell lymphomas arising in the mediastinum. *Journal of Clinical Pathology* **46:** 513–516.

Chan JKC, Ng CS, Hui PK et al (1989) Anaplastic large cell Ki-1 lymphoma. Delineation of two morphological types. *Histopathology* **15:** 11–34.

Chan JKC, Buchanan RF Fletcher CDM (1990) Sarcomatoid variant of anaplastic large-cell Ki-1 lymphoma. *American Journal of Surgical Pathology* **14:** 983–988.

Chan JKC, Banks PM, Cleary ML et al (1994) A proposal for classification of lymphoid neoplasms (by the International Lymphoma Study Group). *Histopathology* **25:** 517–536.

Chott A, Kaserer K, Augustin I et al (1990) Ki-1-positive large cell lymphoma. A clinicopathologic study of 41 cases. *American Journal of Surgical Pathology* **14:** 439–448.

Davey MP, Bongiovanni KF, Kaulfersch W et al (1986) Immunoglobulin and T-cell receptor gene rearrangement and expression in human lymphoid leukemia cells at different stages of maturation. *Proceedings of the National Academy of Sciences of the USA* **83:** 8759–8763.

Deane M, McCarthy KP, Wiedemann LM & Norton JD (1991) An improved method for detection of B lymphoid clonality by PCR. *Leukemia*, **5:** 726–730.

Delsol G, Al Saati T, Gatter KC et al (1988) Coexpression of epithelial membrane antigen (EMA), Ki-1, and interleukin-2 receptor by anaplastic large cell lymphomas. Diagnostic value in so-called malignant histiocytosis. *American Journal of Pathology* **130:** 59–70.

Ford HM, Ridge SH, Cabrera ME et al (1993) in utero rearrangements in the trithorax-related oncogene in infant leuhaemias. *Nature* **363:** 358–360.

Fletcher JA, Lynch EA, Kimball VM et al (1991) Translocation (9;22) is associated with extremely poor prognosis in intensively treated children with acute lymphoblastic leukemia. *Blood* **77:** 435–439.

Frizzera G & Murphy SB (1979) Follicular (nodular) lymphoma in childhood: a rare clinicalpathological entity. *Cancer* **4:** 2218–2235.

Gordon B, Weisenburger D, Warkentin PI et al (1993) Peripheral T-cell lymphoma in childhood and adolescence. A clinicopathologic study of 22 patients. *Cancer* **71:** 257–263.

Greaves M (1993) A natural history for pediatric acute leukemia. *Blood* **82:** 1043–1051.

Greaves MF & Alexander FE (1993) An infectious etiology for common acute lymphoblastic leukemia in childhood? *Leukemia* **7:** 349–360.

Greaves MF, Janossy G, Peto J & Kay H (1981) Immunologically defined subclasses of acute lymphoblastic leukaemia in children: their relationship to presentation features and prognosis. *British Journal of Haematology* **48:** 179–197.

Greaves MF, Pegram SM & Chan LC (1985) Collaborative group study of the epidemiology of acute lymphoblastic leukaemia subtypes: background and first report. *Leukaemia Research* **9:** 715–733.

Greer JP, Kinney MC, Collins RD et al (1991) Clinical features of 31 patients with Ki-1 anaplastic large cell lymphoma *Journal of Clinical Oncology* **9:** 539–547.

Griffith RC, Kelly DR, Nathwani BN et al (1987) A morphologic study of childhood lymphoma of the lymphoblastic type. The Pediatric Oncology Group experience. *Cancer* **59:** 1126–1131.

Grogan TM, Warnke RA & Kaplan HS (1982) A comparative study of Burkitt's and non Burkitt's 'undifferentiated' malignant lymphoma: immunologic, cytochemical, ultrastructural, cytologic, histopathologic, clinical and cell culture features. *Cancer* **49:** 1817–1828.

Herbst H, Tippelmann G, Anagnostopoulos I et al (1989) Immunoglobulin and T-cell receptor gene rearrangements in Hodgkin's Disease and Ki-1-positive anaplastic large cell lymphoma. *Journal of Clinical Oncology* **9:** 539–547.

Hutchison RE, Pui C-H, Murphy SB & Berard CW (1988) Non-Hodgkin's lymphoma in children younger than 3 years. *Cancer* **62:** 1371–1373.

Hutchison RE, Murphy SB, Fairclough DL et al (1989) Diffuse small noncleaved cell lymphoma in children, Burkitt's versus non-Burkitt's types. *Cancer* **64:** 23–28.

Hutchison RE, Fairclough DL, Holt H et al (1991) Clinical significance of histology and immunophenotype in childhood diffuse large cell lymphoma. *Americal Journal of Clinical Pathology* **95:** 787–793.

Isaacson PG, Norton AJ & Addis BJ (1987) The human thymus contains a novel population of B lymphocytes. *Lancet* **ii:** 1488–1491.

Kadin ME, Sako D, Berliner N et al (1986) Childhood Ki-1 lymphoma presenting with skin lesions and peripheral lymphadenopathy. *Blood* **68:** 1042–1049.

Kamps MP, Murre C, Sun X-H & Baltimore D (1990) A new homeobox gene contributes the DNA binding domain of the t(1;19) translocation protein in pre-B ALL. *Cell* **90:** 547–555.

Kaneko Y, Frizzera G, Edamura S et al (1989) A novel translocation t(2;5)(p23;q35) in childhood phagocytic large T-cell lymphoma mimicking malignant histiocytosis. *Blood* **73:** 806–813.

Katz F, Malcolm S, Gibbons B et al (1988) Cellular and molecular studies on infant null acute lymphoblastic leukaemia. *Blood* **71:** 1438–1447.

Kelly DR, Nathwani BN, Griffith RC et al (1987) A morpologic study of childhood lymphoma of the undifferentiated type. The Pediatric Oncology Group experience. *Cancer* **59:** 1132–1137.

Kinney MC, Collins RD, Greer JP et al (1993) A small cell-predominant variant of primary Ki-1 (CD30)+ T-cell lymphoma. *American Journal of Surgical Pathology* **17:** 859–868.

Kitchingman GR, Rovigatti U, Mauer AM et al (1985) Rearrangement of immunoglobulin heavy chain genes in T cell acute lymphoblastic leukemia. *Blood* **65:** 725–729.

Kjeldsberg CR & Wilson JF (1986) Malignant tumours in children. In Finegold M (ed) *Pathology of Neoplasia in Children and Adolescents*, pp 87–125. Philadelphia: W B Saunders.

Kjeldsberg CR, Wilson JF & Berard CW (1983) Non-Hodgkin's lymphoma in chldren. *Human Pathology* **14:** 612–627.

Lamarre L, Jacobson JO, Aisenberg AC & Harris NL (1989) Primary large cell lymphoma of the mediastinum. A histologic and immunophenotypic study of 29 cases. *American Journal of Surgical Pathology* **13:** 730–739.

Leake J, Kellie SJ & Pritchard J (1989) Peripheral T-cell lymphoma in childhood. A clinicopathological study of six cases. *Histopathology* **14:** 255–268.

Le Beau MM, Bitter MA, Larson RA et al (1989) The t(2;5)(p23;q35): a recurring chromosomal abnormality in Ki1-positive anaplastic large cell lymphomas. *Leukaemia* **3:** 866–870.

Lee S-H, Su I-J & Chen R-L (1991) A pathologic study of childhood lymphoma in Taiwan with special reference to peripheral T-cell lymphoma and the association with Epstein–Barr viral infection. *Cancer* **68:** 1954–1962.

Leoncini L, Del Vecchio MT & Kraft R (1990) Hodgkin's disease and CD30-positive anaplastic large cell lymphomas—a continuous spectrum of malignant disorders. *American Journal of Pathology* **137:** 1047–1057.

Lugo TG, Pendergast A-M, Muller AJ & Witte ON (1990) Tyrosine kinase activity and transformation potency of *bcr-abl* oncogene products. *Science* **247:** 1079–1082.

McCarthy KP, Sloane JP & Wiedemann LM (1990) Rapid method for distinguishing clonal from polyclonal B cell populations in surgical biopsy specimens. *Journal of Clinical Pathology* **43:** 429–432.

McCarthy KP, Sloane JP, Kabarowski JHS et al (1991) The rapid detection of clonal T-cell proliferations in patients with lymphoid disorders. *American Journal of Pathology* **138:** 821–828.

McCarthy KP, Sloane JP, Kabarowski JHS et al (1992) A simplified method of detection of clonal rearrangements of the T-cell receptor-γ chain gene. *Diagnostic Molecular Pathology* **1:** 173–179.

McGee J-O'D, Isaacson PG & Wright NA (eds) (1992) *Oxford Textbook of Pathology*, Vol. 2G, Section 30: Diagnostic and Investigative Techniques, pp 2269–2344. Oxford: Oxford University Press.

Magrath IT (1990) The pathogenesis of Burhill Lymphoma. *Advances in Cancer Research* **55:** 133–269.

Mann RB, Jaffe ES, Braylan RC et al (1976) Non-endemic Burkitt's lymphoma: a B cell tumor related to germinal centres. *New England Journal of Medicine* **295:** 685.

Mason DY, Bastard C, Rimokh R et al (1990) CD30-positive large cell lymphomas ('Ki-1 lymphoma') are associated with a chromosomal translocation involving 5q35. *British Journal of Haematology* **74:** 161–168.

Miliauskas JR, Berard CW, Young RC et al (1982) Undifferentiated non-Hodgkin's lymphomas (Burkitt's and non-Burkitt's types). *Cancer* **50:** 2115–2121.

Morgan GJ, Janssen JWG, Guo A-P et al (1989) Polymerase chain reaction for detection of residual leukaemia. *Lancet* **i:** 928–929.

Morgan R, Hecht BK, Sandberg AA & Hecht F (1986) Chromosome 5q35 breakpoint in malignant histiocytosis. *New England Journal of Medicine* **314:** 1322.

Morris SW, Kirstein MN, Valentine MB et al (1994) Fusion of a leinare gene, ALK to a nucleolar protein gene, NPM in non-Hodgkin's lymphome. *Science* **263:** 1281–1284.

Murphy SB (1980) Classification, staging and end results of treatment of childhood non-Hodgkin's lymphomas: dissimilarities from lymphomas in adults. *Seminars in Oncology* **7:** 332–339.

Murphy SB, Fairclough DL, Hutchison RE & Berard CW (1989) Non-Hodgkin's lymphomas of childhood: an analysis of the histology, staging and response to treatment of 338 cases at a single institution. *Journal of Clinical Oncology* **7:** 186–193.

Nathwani BN, Diamond LW, Winberg CD et al (1981) Lymphoblastic lymphoma: a clinicopathologic study of 95 patients. *Cancer* **48:** 234–2357.

Nathwani BN, Griffith RC, Kelly DR et al (1987) A morphologic study of childhood lymphoma of the diffuse 'histiocytic' type. The Pediatric Oncology Group experience. *Cancer* **59:** 1138–1142.

National Cancer Institute (1982) NCI-sponsored study of classification of non-Hodgkin lymphomas. Summary and description of a working formulation for clinical usage. *Cancer* **49:** 2112–2135.

Norton JD, Campana D, Hoffbrand AV et al (1987) Rearrangement of immunoglobulin and T-cell antigen receptor genes in acute myeloid leukaemia with lymphoid-associated markers. *Leukemia* **1:** 757–761.

Nowell PC & Croce CM (1990) Chromosome translocations and oncogenes in human lymphoid tumors. *American Journal of Clinical Pathology* **94:** 229–237.

O'Connor NTJ, Stein H, Gatter KC et al (1987) Genotypic analysis of large cell lymphomas which express the Ki-1 antigen. *Histopathology* **11:** 733–740.

Orscheschek K, Merz H, Hell J et al (1995) Large-cell anaplastic lymphoma—specific translocation (t [2;5] [p23;q35]) in Hogkin's disease: indication of a common pathogenesis? *Lancet* **345:** 87–90.

Pallesen G (1990) The diagnostic significance of the CD30 (Ki-1) antigen. *Histopathology* **16:** 409–413.

Pébasque MJ, Lafage-Pochitaloff M, Gallard F et al (1993) Localization of two tyrosine kinase receptor genes with respect to the 5q 35 chromosomal break point of Ki-1 lymphoma cell lines. *Genes, Chromosomes and Cancer* **8:** 119–126.

Perrone T, Frizzera G & Rosai J (1986) Mediastinal diffuse large-cell lymphoma with sclerosis. A clinicopathologic study of 60 cases. *American Journal of Surgical Pathology* **10:** 176–191.

Pileri S, Falini B, Delsol G et al (1990) Lymphohistiocytic T-cell lymphoma (anaplastic large cell lymphoma CD30+/Ki-1 + with a high content of reactive histiocytes). *Histopathology* **16:** 383–391.

Piris M, Brown DC, Gatter KC & Mason DY (1990) CD30 expression in non-Hodgkin's lymphoma. *Histopathology* **17:** 211–218.

Piris M, Gatter KC & Mason DY (1991) CD30 expression in follicular lymphoma. *Histopathology* **18:** 25–29.

Potter MN, Cross NCP, van Dongen JJM et al (1993) Molecular evidence of minimal residual disease after treatment for leukaemia and lymphoma: an updated meeting report and review. *Leukemia* **7:** 1302–1314.

Pui C-H, Williams DL, Raimondi SC et al (1987) Hypodiploidy is associated with a poor prognosis in childhood acute lymphoblastic leukemia. *Blood* **70:** 247–253.

Pui C–H, Carroll AJ, Head D et al (1990a) Near-triploid and near-tetraploid acute lymphoblastic leukemia of childhood. *Blood* **76:** 590–596.

Pui CH, Carroll AJ, Raimondi SC et al (1990b) Clinical presentation, karyotypic characterisation and treatment outcome of childhood acute lymphoblastic leukaemia with a near-haploid or hypodiploid < 45 line. *Blood* **75:** 1170–1177.

Pui C-H, Frankel LS, Carroll AJ et al (1991) Clinical characteristics and treatment outcome of childhood acute lymphoblastic leukemia with the t(4; 11)(q21; q23): a collaborative study of 40 cases. *Blood* **71:** 440–447.

Raimondi SC, Peiper SC, Kitchingman GR et al (1989) Childhood acute lymphoblastic leukemia with chromosomal breakpoints at 11q23. *Blood* **73:** 1627–1634.

Raimondi SC, Behm FG, Roberson PK et al (1990) Cytogenetics of pre-B-cell acute lymphoblastic leukemia with emphasis on prognostic implications of the t(1;19). *Journal of Clinical Oncology* **8:** 1380–1388.

Ribeiro RC, Pui C-H & Murphy SB (1992) Childhood malignant non-Hodgkin lymphomas of uncommon histology. *Leukemia* **6:** 761–765.

Rimokh R, Magand J-P, Berger F et al (1989) A translocation involving a specific breakpoint (q35) on chromosome 5 is characteristic of anaplastic large cell lymphoma (Ki-1 lymphoma) *British Journal of Haematology* **71:** 31–36.

Rovigatti U, Mirro J, Kitchingman G et al (1984) Heavy chain immunoglobulin gene rearrangement in acute nonlymphocytic leukemia. *Blood* **63:** 1023–1027.

Rowley JD (1990) Recurring chromosome abnormalities in leukemia and lymphoma. *Seminars in Haematology* **27:** 122–136.

Schnitzer B, Roth MS, Hyder DM & Ginsburg D (1988) Ki-1 lymphomas in children. *Cancer* **61:** 1213–1221.

Schwab U, Stein H, Gerdes J et al (1982) Production of a monoclonal antibody specific for Hodgkin and Sternberg–Reed cells of Hodgkin's disease and a subset of normal lymphoid cells. *Nature* **299:** 65–67.

Secker-Walker LM, Chessells JM, Stewart EL et al (1989) Chromosomes and other prognostic factors in acute lymphoblastic leukaemia: a long-term follow-up. *British Journal of Haematology* **72:** 336–342.

Shikano T, Kaneko Y, Takazawa M et al (1986) Balanced and unbalanced 1; 19 translocation associated acute lymphoblastic leukemias. *Cancer* **58:** 2239–2243.

Southern EM (1975) Detection of specific sequences among DNA fragments separated by gel electrophoresis. *Journal of Molecular Biology* **98:** 503–517.

Stansfeld AG, Diebold J, Kapanci Y et al (1988) Updated Kiel classification for lymphomas. *Lancet* **i:** 292–293.

Stein H, Mason DY, Gerdes J et al (1985) The expression of the Hodgkin's disease associated antigen Ki-1 in reactive and neoplastic lymphoid tissue: evidence that Reed–Sternberg cells and histiocytic malignancies are derived from activated lymphoid cells. *Blood* **66:** 848–858.
Vecchi V, Burnelli R, Pileri S et al (1993) Anaplastic large cell lymphoma (Ki-1 +/CD30+) in childhood. *Medical and Pediatric Oncology* **21:** 402–410.
Wilson JF, Jenkin RDT, Anderson JR et al (1984) Studies on the pathology of non-Hodgkin's lymphoma of childhood. I. The role of routine histopathology as a prognostic factor. A report from the Childrens Cancer Study Group. *Cancer* **53:** 1695–1704.
Wilson JF, Kjeldsberg CR, Sposto R et al (1987) The pathology of non-Hodgkin's lymphoma of childhood: II. Reproducibility and relevance of the histologic classification of 'undifferentiated' lymphomas (Burkitt's versus non-Burkitt's). *Human Pathology* **18:** 1008–1014.
Winberg CD, Nathwani BN, Bearman RM & Rappaport H (1981) Follicular (nodular) lymphoma during the first two decades of life: a clinicopathologic study of 12 patients. *Cancer* **48:** 222–235.
World Health Organization, Geneva (1969) Histopathological definition of Burkitt's tumour.
Yano T, van Keiken HJM, Magrath IT et al (1992) Histogenetic correlations between subcategories of small noncleaved cell lymphomas. *Blood* **79:** 1282–1290.
Ziemin-van der Poel S, McCabe NR, Gill HJ et al (1991) Identification of a gene, MLL, that spans the breakpoint in 11q23 translocations associated with human leukemias. *Proceedings of the National Academy of Sciences of the USA* **88:** 10 735–10 739.

3

Infectious complications of treatment

T. R. ROGERS

Infectious complications have persisted as a major cause of morbidity throughout the evolution of treatment for childhood haematological malignancies. Yet the good remission rates achieved today are at least partly due to more effective protocols for prevention and management of infection. Many of these protocols are based on experience gained from the treatment of adults and then adapted for the paediatric setting. It should be remembered that common childhood infections, often due to viruses, may present in more severe form during cancer chemotherapy. However, the principal infections seen are due to the now well recognized opportunistic pathogens.

Better survival has facilitated the use of more intensive chemotherapy regimens. To some extent the prolongation of profound neutropenia that might be anticipated as a consequence can now be prevented by use of recombinant haemopoietic growth factors (Gisselbrecht et al, 1994), so that infections complicating acute immunosuppression can be contained. However, chemotherapy given over more prolonged time periods for consolidation, and treatment by bone marrow transplantation, are likely to lead to a more persistent state of immune suppression, an extended spectrum of opportunistic infections over and above those frequently seen during neutropenia and a less predictable clinical presentation. Some of these late infections, such as pneumococcal sepsis, can be rapidly fatal and need to be anticipated.

It should also be borne in mind that infection is a common initial presentation in children with acute leukaemia or lymphoma, and it needs aggressive treatment if possible before beginning immunosuppressive therapy.

THE NATURE OF IMMUNOLOGICAL DEFECTS IN LEUKAEMIA AND LYMPHOMA

It is a traditional view that the defects in host immunity to infection caused by acute leukaemia are associated primarily with both quantitative and qualitative deficiencies of neutrophils resulting in a particular association with bacterial sepsis, while in lymphomas the effects of the disease on

Baillière's Clinical Paediatrics—
Vol. 3, No. 4, November 1995
ISBN 0–7020–2075–3

cellular immunity account for susceptibility to intracellular bacterial, fungal and viral pathogens (Young, 1994). However this fails to take adequate account of the potentially immunosuppressive effect of the various treatment regimens currently employed.

The acute consequence of chemotherapy in either disease is the rapid onset of profound neutropenia, and current more intensive regimens are leading to the risk of prolonged periods before bone marrow recovery. Additionally there is almost invariably a breach of the mucosal defences consequent upon cytotoxic chemotherapy with mucositis (Childers et al, 1993) which facilitates bacterial invasion from the oropharynx and intestinal tract.

Consolidation treatment may be immunosuppressive and may be associated with further periods of neutropenia with the attendant risk of late bacterial or fungal infections, or, if steroids are being given on a prolonged basis, the likelihood of infection with intracellular pathogens or *Pneumocystis carinii* will be significantly greater.

Children undergoing BMT will additionally have defective T-cell function concurrent with a risk of irradiation-induced damage to the lungs which significantly increase the severity of viral pnemonias. Late infections are in some cases due to defective humoral immune responses and the inability to opsonize and phagocytose pneumococci and *Haemophilus influenzae*. This may simply be due to quantitative deficiencies of immunoglobulins but more specifically can be related to low levels of IgG subclasses e.g. IgG2 (Rogers et al, 1986); furthermore, hyposplenism or asplenia, if present, is associated with a deficiency of opsonizing antibodies to these pyogenic organisms.

STRATEGIES FOR THE MANAGEMENT OF INFECTION

At presentation of disease

An acute bacterial infection may be the presenting feature of the underlying disease, but even when this is not the case the patient should be carefully screened for evidence of occult infection which might be exacerbated by subsequent treatment. This includes a careful physical and dental examination, chest and sinus X-rays, throat, stool and urine cultures. A base-line serum sample is necessary for subsequent antibody tests, as well as for determining CMV serological status in allogeneic transplant recipients.

Prevention of infection during neutropenia

The strategies employed here are broadly divided into, firstly, chemoprophylaxis to prevent endogenously acquired bacterial and fungal infections and, secondly, protected environments to prevent exogenously acquired infection with airborne fungal pathogens such as *Aspergillus* (see Table 1).

Table 1. Measures to prevent infection during remission-induction chemotherapy or bone marrow transplantation.

Before treatment	Full physical examination Immunization history Chest and nasal sinus X-rays Throat, stool, urine cultures Base-line serum e.g. for CMV antibody[a] Insertion of indwelling catheter with aseptic precautions
During neutropenia	Chemoprophylaxis: Co-trimoxazole + colistin Fluconazole *or* itraconozole[b] Chlorhexidine mouth gargles Single-room isolation (HEPA-filtered room for 'high-risk' patients[a]) 'Clean' food diet Limited weekly surveillance cultures e.g. throat, stool, catheter exit site
After marrow recovery/engraftment	Chemoprophylaxis: Co-trimoxazole → 12 months[a] Penicillin[c] Itraconazole[c] Immunization: see Table 3 Advice on dietary items to avoid e.g. salads

[a] BMT patients.
[b] See text.
[c] In the presence of immunosuppression for GHD.

Many of our existing protocols are rooted in this traditional approach to prevention of infection in the neutropenic patient, but need constant re-appraisal in order to ensure their current appropriateness.

Numerous comparisons have been made between different prophylactic antibiotic regimens to establish their efficacy (Vossen et al, 1990; Donnelly et al, 1992). These have included a combination of the oral non-absorbed agents neomycin, colistin and nystatin, the systemically absorbed co-trimoxazole and, more recently, fluoroquinolones such as ciprofloxacin, or norfloxacin.

In summary, it can be concluded that each of these regimens significantly reduces the incidence of intercurrent bacterial infections due to Gram-negative rods such as *Escherichia coli* and *Proteus* by virtue of their suppressive effects on the intestinal flora. However, more widespread use as a result of their success may be a factor in the emergence of resistant Gram-positive bacteria which have become the predominant cause of sepsis during neutropenia. These can be further subdivided into the coagulase-negative staphylococci, mostly originating from the skin and probably gaining access to the blood via tunnelled intravascular catheters, and viridans streptococci, originating from the oropharynx—especially in patients with mucositis. Unfortunately there are no antibiotics that can provide cover for this spectrum of potential pathogens and be safely given throughout neutropenia. Many of the viridans streptococci are penicillin-resistant, while the coagulase-negative staphylococci are often multiply antibiotic-resistant.

The quinolones provide the best systemic protection against Gram-negative infection as they include in their spectrum *Pseudomonas aeruginosa* which is not covered by the other antimicrobials. This is important because this organism still accounts for the highest morbidity when causing septicaemia. However, fear of damage to growing cartilage, based on early toxicity studies in beagle dogs, has prevented the quinolones being licensed for use in children.

Measures to prevent streptococcal infection have focused on ensuring good oral hygiene and reducing the incidence of mucositis.

Herpes simplex virus is an important cause of oral mucositis. Even though the prevalence of seropositivity to this virus, as an indicator of latent infection, is likely to be low in children, the use of prophylactic acyclovir should be considered in seropositive children because it significantly reduces the incidence of herpes mucositis.

Infections continue to frequently complicate the use of intravascular catheters; indeed the rate at which these occur is reported to be higher in children than in adults (Darbyshire et al, 1985; Barnes and Rogers, 1987). The most effective preventive strategy is likely to develop from a better understanding of the pathogenesis of these infections. Tunnelled catheters should be inserted by an operator experienced in this procedure. Aseptic precautions should be taken. There is no evidence to support the administration of a prophylactic antibiotic such as vancomycin at the time of insertion. A breach in the skin that is inevitable with Hickman catheters is most likely to provide the route by which local or systemic infection occurs. Evidence is available to suggest that the frequency of manipulation of the catheter is important in determining the rate of infection. Also, it has been found that triple-lumen catheters cause a higher rate of infection than single-lumen ones. Aseptic precautions when handling the catheter for a procedure are likely to reduce the chances of colonization of the catheter hub and the risk of infection. For long-term use, implantable ports appear to be less likely to become infected compared with Hickman or Broviac catheters (Mirro et al, 1990).

Approaches to preventing fungal infections have paralleled those used for bacterial prophylaxis. Although the orally administered polyenes nystatin and amphotericin B can suppress colonizing yeasts in the intestinal tract, they are not absorbed and therefore offer no systemic protection against fungal infection. The new triazole antifungals, fluconazole and itraconazole, therefore represent a significant improvement over the polyenes since they are absorbed systemically after oral administration. Fluconazole has been evaluated in several recent comparative trials of prophylaxis and been found to provide protection against both mucosal and invasive candidiasis, with only few mild drug-related side-effects being observed. However, there are concerns over the limited antifungal spectrum of this drug since in the case of the neutropenic patient it is reliably active only against *Candida albicans* and *Candida tropicalis* (which together cause $>80\%$ of candida infections) while some of the emerging species such as *Candida glabrata* and *Candida krusei* are likely to be resistant (Wingard et al, 1991); furthermore, there is now clear evidence in vivo that *Aspergillus* spp are resistant as well.

Published data on the efficacy of itraconazole as a prophylactic agent are, by contrast, relatively limited. The absorption of any of the currently licensed formulations of the drug from the gastrointestinal tract is poor when the patient is receiving H2 receptor antagonists or when gastric acid production is impaired for whatever reason. However, its spectrum of activity includes more species of *Candida* than fluconazole and, notably, *Aspergillus*. Problems with bio-availability are likely to have been overcome with the development of a cyclodextrin formulation (Prentice et al, 1994), and this is currently the subject of clinical trial evaluation. It is appropriate to administer antifungal prophylaxis where there is the prospect of neutropenia for 2 weeks or longer. In patients who are receiving remission induction chemotherapy fluconazole is an appropriate choice because *C. albicans* and *C. tropicalis* are the main pathogenic species concerned (Marina et al, 1991). However, itraconazole is recommended for transplant recipients, those with prolonged bone marrow failure (neutropenia > 3 weeks), and in children with a previous history of aspergillosis who are undergoing further immunosuppressive therapy (Turner et al, 1993; Cowie et al, 1994).

It is acknowledged that some clinicians and microbiologists elect not to give any chemoprophylaxis during neutropenia on the basis that infection in their patients is infrequent and because the use of antimicrobials will encourage selection of resistant bacteria and yeasts. While there is some justification for this view in units treating patients with low risk of infection, there is nevertheless overwhelming evidence in favour of prophylaxis where there is a higher risk of infection. To some extent this will depend on individual units' past experience and on how well they are able to document infections.

Protected environments

A well established part of the preventive strategy during neutropenia is single-room isolation of the patient, thereby providing a physical barrier from fellow patients. While nursing the patient this will normally involve the donning of masks and aprons by attendant staff, restricting food items to those with minimal bacterial and fungal counts, and limiting the number of visitors entering the room. These measures may be described as prudent rather than having proven efficacy. Staff or relatives with symptoms of upper respiratory tract infection should not come into contact with the patient. Rooms that filter the air prior to entry and maintain positive pressure and a high rate of air circulation will yield significantly reduced bacterial and fungal spore counts and have been found to reduce the incidence of aspergillosis in high-risk BMT patients (Barnes and Rogers, 1989). These are expensive facilities and are likely to be cost-effective only in allogeneic bone marrow transplant recipients in whom the risk of aspergillosis is greatest. Some of these patients may already be harbouring *Aspergillus* in nasal sinus or upper respiratory tract as a result of previous immunosuppressive chemotherapy, in which case they will receive no benefit from filtered air. Nevertheless it can be concluded that, in the paediatric patient, physical segregation from other similarly ill children, in a single room, will reduce the incidence of intercurrent bacterial and viral infections.

One of the clostridia, *Clostridium difficile*, is recognized to be a nosocomial pathogen in immunocompromised hosts, and clustering of cases on a transplant unit has been reported (Rogers et al, 1981). *C. difficile* toxin-induced diarrhoea is a complication of the effects of antibiotics on the intestinal flora which can be treated with metronidazole; however, prevention of cross-infection with this organism is dependent on staff having knowledge of both its mode of transmission and the value of good handwashing technique. Nosocomially acquired viruses such as rotavirus and small round structured viruses (e.g. Norwalk agent) are principally transmitted in the same way and may cause outbreaks of vomiting and diarrhoea. The use of antiseptic handwashes or rubs containing chlorhexidine is probably of value in high-risk units as a more effective way for removing contaminating viruses. A further possible cause of diarrhoea is *Cryptosporidium parvum*. The organism can be demonstrated in the stools by a modified Ziehl–Neelsen stain. Clustering of cases on a leukaemia unit, with some patients suffering from persistent diarrhoea, has been reported (Foot et al, 1990).

MANAGEMENT OF THE FEBRILE NEUTROPENIC CHILD

Empirical antibiotic therapy

In a neutropenic patient the development of fever of 38°C or greater is usually taken to indicate the likelihood of infection and the necessity for empirical therapy. Prior to starting treatment a full physical examination should be made, with special attention being given to any pulmonary or cutaneous abnormalities as these are often the sites where infection is first evident; this includes inspection of the indwelling catheter site for signs of local infection. At least two blood culture sets should be taken initially and, in addition, samples from any suspected foci such as the urinary tract. X-rays of the chest or other sites will be performed as indicated (see Table 2).

Prompt initiation of broad-spectrum antibiotic therapy is necessary primarily to cover the possibility of Gram-negative septicaemia since this causes the greatest morbidity. Cover against *Pseudomonas aeruginosa* is therefore mandatory, even in patients who may have been receiving ciprofloxacin prophylaxis since quinolone-resistant strains have been reported in such circumstances. Different empirical antibiotic regimens have been evaluated over the years, the results of which lead to the conclusion that the combination of a broad-spectrum penicillin with an aminoglycoside, e.g. piperacillin and gentamicin, or, monotherapy with ceftazidime, produce the best response rates with a very low incidence of fatal infections. On average, fever will take 4 days to settle when antibiotics are appropriate to the infection. However, it is now clear that, with the high incidence of staphylococcal bacteraemias, many of which are catheter-associated, fever will often not respond to these antibiotics and a change to a more effective agent will be necessary. Either vancomycin or teicoplanin will be appropriate here. There has been considerable debate over whether it would be better to give vancomycin in the initial therapy regimen, but the consensus view is that this is not necessary or desirable because, firstly, infections with coagulase-negative staphylococci are not rapidly fatal in the way that Gram-negative infections can be and, secondly, glycopeptides are potentially ototoxic and should be used very selectively; a further issue is the role of glycopeptide use in encouraging the emergence of resistant enterococci which have been reported from haematology units where glycopeptide usage is high. It therefore seems that these agents can be started when there is persistent fever in spite of the initial antibiotic regimen or when staphylococci have been recovered from blood cultures, or both.

Table 2. Approach to management of suspected infection during neutropenia.

Initial investigations	Full physical examination Chest X-ray, CT scan as indicated Blood, urine cultures Throat, urine cultures for CMV or other viruses[a]
Initial empirical therapy	Piperacillin and gentamicin, or ceftazidime
Adjustment for persistent fever	
Fever at 48–96 hours	Add vancomycin or teicoplanin
at 5–7 days	Add amphotericin B
Further investigations	Bronchoalveolar lavage in the presence of pulmonary infiltrates Fungal antigen tests on serum or urine[b]
Continue therapy until	Patient afebrile for 7 days and no infection documented Marrow recovery or longer in case of documented infection[c]

[a] BMT patients.
[b] Still experimental.
[c] See text for details.

In cases of vascular catheter-associated sepsis a common question is: should the line be removed? Generally this should not be necessary since many coagulase-negative staphylococci infections respond fully to antibiotics (Uderzo et al, 1992). Exceptions are Gram-negative and fungal line sepsis where the recommendation is to change the catheter under appropriate antibiotic cover.

It is clear that, in many episodes of neutropenic fever, no microbial cause is ever documented. The pathogenesis of fever in these cases is an area for further study since this would help to rationalize on antibiotic treatment. In neutropenic BMT recipients graft-versus-host disease (GVHD) is another possible cause of fever. There may be signs of cutaneous GVHD but, if not, there are some laboratory tests that may help in distinguishing this from infection—such as measurement of the acute-phase reactants C-reactive protein (elevated in bacterial infection) (Walker et al, 1984) and neopterin (elevated in GVHD) (Sheldon et al, 1991).

The duration of antibiotic therapy should be dictated by the speed of response of the fever, whether a pathogen has been isolated, and the neutrophil count. In a case where the fever responds promptly and no pathogen is identified, a 7-day course of treatment may be adequate even in the face of persisting neutropenia. This contrasts with the situation where a pathogen has been isolated, the patient is systemically unwell, and profound neutropenia is likely to persist for several days. Here, continuation of antibiotics until fever has fully resolved and marrow recovery has occurred is justified, especially where the cause is Gram-negative sepsis.

Empirical antifungal therapy

Fever persisting for 5 days or longer in the face of appropriate empirical antibiotic therapy raises the possibility of opportunistic fungal infection, due most likely to *Candida* or *Aspergillus*. Even in the absence of localized signs of infection it is standard practice to administer antifungal therapy at this point on the basis that fungal infection is very likely in a persistently febrile patient who continues to be profoundly neutropenic (Barnes and Rogers, 1988), and because any delay will allow the infection to become established with the likelihood of a high morbidity (Pizzo et al, 1982).

Amphotericin B continues to be the agent of first choice because of its broad spectrum of activity. Of the other possible choices for this role, fluconazole would be contra-indicated if the patient had been receiving it for prophylaxis but also, as mentioned earlier, there is concern that it has a narrower spectrum of antifungal activity. At present itraconazole can be given only orally, with uncertainty over its absorption, so that it is not ideally suited to this role either.

Signs in support of a diagnosis of fungal infection include pulmonary infiltrates, skin lesions, sudden deterioration of hepatic function or development of neurological signs. Appropriate investigations would be bronchoscopy and lavage, CT scan of lungs, liver or brain according to the suspected site of infection. Biopsy of a skin lesion or other organ may be justified when faced with a patient who is deteriorating and in whom the diagnosis has not been established. Further justification for an aggressive approach to diagnosis is the emergence of new fungal pathogens such as *Fusarium*, *Pseudoallescheria boydii* or hyphomycetes, some of which respond poorly to amphotericin B and where other therapies may be more appropriate (Rogers, 1994). Non-culture methods of detecting fungi have been evaluated in severely immunocompromised patients and have shown promise; these include fungal antigen detection (Rogers et al, 1990) and amplification of fungal DNA in blood, urine, bronchoalveolar lavage (Tang et al, 1993) or other body fluids. If proved reliable these tests could be employed to predict which patients are likely to progress to invasive fungal infection, thereby enabling early therapy to be given with greater confidence. Antifungal therapy should be continued until at least 7 days after the fever has responded in a case where no pathogen is isolated and where the index of suspicion for fungal infection is low. For treatment of a documented fungal infection this will depend on the pathogen involved and the patient's neutrophil count. In cases of candidaemia, 2 to 4 weeks of treatment may suffice when bone marrow recovery has occurred and any vascular catheters implicated have been removed. In contrast, at least 6 weeks of treatment is recommended where there is evidence of deep organ involvement by *Candida*, and also in cases of aspergillosis.

A frequent problem that arises when giving 'conventional' amphotericin B is nephrotoxicity as this can be reversed only by stopping the drug. It is now possible to overcome this problem by administering a lipid-based formulation of the drug of which there are now three available and licensed in the UK for this indication. One approach is to switch when the serum creatinine rises to 140 µmol/l following which an improvement in renal function can be anticipated. Experience to date has confirmed the kidney-sparing properties of these formulations but there is as yet no evidence to show that any of them is more effective than conventional amphotericin B. Randomized trials comparing liposomal amphotericin B (Ambisome) with the parent drug are currently under way (I. M. Hann, personal communication).

For the treatment of aspergillosis itraconazole should be considered as an alternative to amphotericin B in view of its good activity in vitro against the causative organism and reports of clinical success (Moore et al, 1993). Only the cyclodextrin formulation should be used so as to ensure therapeutic tissue concentrations; clearly, its use will depend on the patient being able to take and tolerate oral medication. An intravenous formulation of this drug is about to be evaluated for clinical efficacy. There are no data to support combining amphotericin B with an azole such as itraconazole in aspergillosis; but there is some in vitro evidence to suggest that under certain circumstances they may be antagonistic. The role of surgery for resection of a pulmonary aspergilloma in a neutropenic patient is uncertain although there are some reports of success with this approach in adults (H.G. Prentice, personal communication).

The use of growth factors as an adjunct to antimicrobial therapy of documented infection during neutropenia has been studied (Bodey et al, 1994) but the results are too preliminary to make a recommendation.

INFECTIONS COMPLICATING BONE MARROW TRANSPLANTATION

Specific groups of infections are recognized as being common at different time periods after allogeneic BMT (Rogers and Selwyn, 1994). Those infections associated with the neutropenic period have been dealt with in the previous section.

Following engraftment, the principal opportunistic pathogens are cytomegalovirus (CMV) and *Pneumocystis carinii* (Bowden and Meyers, 1994). CMV pneumonia has been recognized over the past decade to be the major infective cause of mortality in BMT. Risk factors include CMV seropositivity in the transplant recipient and development of GVHD requiring immunosuppressive therapy. In children the prevalence of CMV antibody, as an indicator of latent infection, is considerably lower than in adults. There is, however, a risk of transmitting the virus in unscreened transfused blood products resulting in primary infection in a seronegative recipient. The principal clinical manifestation of disease due to CMV infection is interstitial pneumonia. The diagnosis is established by demonstrating the presence of CMV early antigen in bronchoalveolar lavage. Combination of ganciclovir with high-titre CMV immunoglobulin is the treatment of choice. Screening of donors, so that only seronegative blood products are given to seronegative transplant patients, has proven to be very effective in reducing the incidence of pneumonia (Bowden et al, 1987). In seropositive adult patients pre-emptive therapy with ganciclovir in response to evidence of virus reactivation has been found to reduce the incidence of CMV pneumonia (Schmidt et al, 1991). Patients undergoing intensive chemotherapy followed by autologous transplantation are likely to have a low incidence of CMV pneumonia. The incidence in recipients of stem cell transplants has yet to be clearly determined.

Human herpes virus 6 is now recognized to be the cause of roseola infantum, but appears also to be a cause of pneumonia after BMT that has many features in common with CMV pneumonia (Cone et al, 1993). It has also been reported to cause an infectious mononucleosis-like illness in immunocompromised individuals. The virus is susceptible to both ganciclovir and foscarnet but is resistant to acyclovir. Adenoviruses and respiratory syncytial virus (Hertz et al, 1989) have also been documented as causes of pneumonia after transplantation.

Pneumocystis carinii can similarly cause life-threatening interstitial pneumonia during the same time period after BMT, but because this is most likely to occur as a complication of latent infection the incidence can be expected to be lower in children than in adults. Chemoprophylaxis with trimethoprim–sulphamethoxazole given at engraftment and continued for 1 year post-transplant has proven highly effective. Trimethoprim alone is not effective. This should be given irrespective of serological status since there is a continuing risk of exposure to the organism via the respiratory route.

Late infections occur beyond 3 months post-transplant and are a consequence of delayed immune reconstitution. The principal opportunistic pathogens are varicella zoster virus usually presenting as shingles, and capsulate strains of *Streptococcus pneumoniae* and *Haemophilus influenzae* causing pneumonia and septicaemia. Overwhelming pneumococcal infection may also complicate asplenia, hyposplenism or immunoglobulin deficiencies associated with GVHD after transplantation. The patients who are most susceptible to infection are likely to respond least well to the pneumococcal vaccine, and this alone cannot be relied upon to provide protection. The *H. influenzae*-type tetanus conjugate vaccine appears by contrast to be more effective in inducing a protective immune response even in the presence of GVHD and has been recommended for both allogeneic and autologous BMT recipients (Ljungman et al, 1995). In addition, prophylactic penicillin should be given to provide protection against pneumococcus; currently, the prevalence of pneumococcal resistance to penicillin in the UK is less than 2% so that this is not a major concern in this context.

Immunization after BMT

For long-term survivors of both allogeneic and autologous BMT immunization can be recommended because of the loss of protective immunity that may be a consequence of the transplant. The European Group for Blood and Marrow Transplantation infectious diseases working party have recently made recommendations on this subject as follows (see Table 3). A firm recommendation is made to vaccinate with killed poliovirus and influenza virus vaccines, diphtheria and tetanus toxoids, and against *H. influenzae* and hepatitis B virus. By contrast, vaccination is generally not recommended with live attenuated virus vaccines against e.g. measles, rubella or mumps and, more specifically, is contra-indicated in patients with chronic GVHD (Ljungman et al, 1995).

Table 3. Recommendations for active immunization of children with haematological malignancy.

Bone marrow transplant recipients not receiving immunosuppression at 12 months[a]	*Strongly recommended* Tetanus toxoid Diphtheria toxoid Inactivated polio Influenza *Recommended* Hepatitis B[b] *H. influenzae* *Not generally recommended* Measles, mumps, rubella Pneumococcus
Patients receiving chemotherapy[c]	Hepatitis B[b] Pneumococcus

[a] Adapted from Ljungman et al (1995).
[b] Ideally, donor and recipient should be immunized before transplant, especially in regions of high endemicity for hepatitis B.
[c] In addition to childhood immunizations being up-to-date.

OTHER INFECTIONS ASSOCIATED WITH CHRONIC IMMUNOSUPPRESSION

Varicella-zoster

A primary infection with varicella-zoster virus results in chickenpox and is usually followed by life-long immunity to this disease, so that when an immunosuppressed child who has a history of having had chickenpox is exposed to a case this should not pose a threat of re-infection or the need for action. The exception would be a child exposed while recovering from a BMT where immunity may have been abolished; in such a case prophylactic acyclovir may be justified. Chickenpox in the immunocompromised is a potentially life-threatening infection because of the high risk of dissemination of the virus to the lungs, causing pneumonitis, brain, liver or skin (Chen et al, 1994). Therefore, a child with haematological malignancy and no previous history of chickenpox who has contact with a case should be given varicella-zoster immuneglobulin (VZIG) at the earliest opportunity but no later than 96 hours after exposure for it to be effective (Centers for Disease Control, 1984). VZIG may not prevent the development of chickenpox but it should reduce the severity of the infection if acquired.

Immunocompromised children who develop shingles as a result of reactivation of the virus also are at increased risk of dissemination of the virus and therefore need prompt treatment with acyclovir. Immunological reconstitution and effective immunity to VZV after BMI may take a year or longer to develop (Takaue et al, 1994) which probably explains the frequency of shingles as a late complication.

A live attenuated VZV vaccine has been carefully studied and found to be safe and immunogenic in children with malignant diseases (Gerson et al, 1984) providing it is not given while the child is receiving active immunosuppression (Brunell et al, 1982). In an attempt to reduce the risk of household exposure to VZV, Diaz et al (1991) gave the vaccine to sibling contacts of children with haematological malignancy. None of the susceptible children developed infection with the vaccine strain or developed chickenpox. However, three of four vaccinees who subsequently had a mild breakthrough infection transmitted to their susceptible sibling. In conclusion, VZV vaccine has been shown to produce good immunity in leukaemic children with few side-effects, although some break-through infections do occur which may require antiviral therapy. The incidence of reactivation infection and development of shingles in vaccinees is no greater than that in children with a history of natural chickenpox (Lawrence et al, 1988). Therefore, vaccination can be recommended in this group. However, this has not been practised in the UK to date, perhaps because of fears of giving a live virus vaccine to an immunocompromised patient. Preference is given to passive immunization on exposure and acyclovir use as indicated above.

Measles

This is another potentially life threatening infection in the immunocompromised child. Following the widespread uptake of the MMR triple vaccine, the number of children with haematological malignancy who are non-immune should progressively decrease. However, those children not previously vaccinated are susceptible to this highly infectious virus. The initial clinical presentation of fever and the typical rash may progress to development of interstitial 'giant cell' pneumonia (Siegel et al, 1977); in some of these cases there may be no preceding rash (Pullan et al, 1976). Measles itself is immunosuppressive and can be complicated by secondary bacterial pneumonia. Encephalitis is the other major complication and can take weeks or months to develop after the initial infection.

There is no specific treatment for measles. Ribavirin aerosol may be considered in cases of pneumonia. Steroids appear to have no useful role. Passive immunization with 'normal' immunoglobulin should be given to an immunocompromised child who is exposed to measles even though its protective efficacy is not established.

Parvovirus infection

Human parvovirus B19 is the causative agent of erythema infectiosum, an infectious disease of childhood presenting with a rash but which may be complicated by marrow aplasia or haemolytic anaemia (Kurtzman et al, 1988). It is normally transmitted by the respiratory route but can also be acquired from blood transfusion. In immunocompromised children, including those with leukaemia, it can cause a severe chronic anaemia. Diagnosis is made by demonstrating parvovirus IgM in serum and finding abnormal red cell precursors in the bone marrow. Administration of intravenous immunoglobulin may produce clinical remission (Koch et al, 1990).

Hepatitis

The risk of becoming infected with hepatitis B or C viruses is increased in patients with haematological malignancy as a consequence of multiple transfusions of blood or blood products. There is therefore an increased likelihood of chronic liver disease in this group (Fink et al, 1993). In addition to the screening of donors for virus carriers before transfusion, hepatitis B vaccine can be offered to patients. Rokicka-Milewska et al (1993) found that most of their children with leukaemia or lymphoma who were not receiving chemotherapy produced a lasting protective antibody response to a course of immunization, whereas those receiving maintenance chemotherapy did not do so.

BACTERIAL, FUNGAL AND OTHER INFECTIONS ASSOCIATED WITH CHRONIC IMMUNOSUPPRESSION

There is a small group of opportunistic pathogens that have a particular predilection for patients receiving long-term immunosuppression. These include the bacteria *Nocardia asteroides*, *Mycobacterium tuberculosis* and *Listeria monocytogenes*, the fungi *Cryptococcus neoformans* and *Aspergillus fumigatus*, and the protozoan *Toxoplasma gondii*.

Children developing chest symptoms with pulmonary infection should be aggressively investigated for possible tuberculosis. Those with a history of previous tuberculous infection or recent exposure to a case of 'open' tuberculosis should be given prophylactic isoniazid. Nocardia infection typically presents as pulmonary abscesses, but the organism may cause bacteraemia or brain abscesses in addition. Co-trimoxazole is the treatment of choice.

With the development of meningitis symptoms in a child with lymphoma or leukaemia, listeriosis and cryptococcosis should be considered as possible diagnoses. *Listeria monocytogenes* causes an acute bacterial meningitis but also cerebritis sometimes progressing to brain abscess. The organism may also be grown from blood cultures. Ampicillin is the drug of choice for treatment. *Cryptococcus neoformans* causes a more insidious form of meningitis with a lymphocytic response in the cerebrospinal fluid.

Cryptococcal antigen is a useful test for diagnosis and exclusion of this infection. Amphotericin B or fluconazole should be equally effective therapy.

Toxoplasma gondii causes a systemic infection but there is a predilection for the central nervous system with either focal lesions, often involving the basal ganglia, or encephalitis. Pyrimethamine plus sulphonamide is treatment of first choice. For further details of these infections see Rogers (1990).

SUMMARY

Opportunistic infection is a well recognized complication of childhood haematological malignancy. Most infections arise as a result of intensive remission–induction therapy and may be bacterial, fungal or viral in aetiology. In recent years the use of more effective broad-spectrum antibiotics has reduced morbidity due to bacterial infection, while fungi have emerged as the major infective cause of death during neutropenia.

Algorithms can be useful in managing infections and include both preventive and therapeutic strategies. In high-risk marrow transplant recipients, protected environments may have a beneficial role in preventing nosocomial aspergillosis. Chronic immunosuppression with steroids increases the risk of infection due to intracellular pathogens. Central nervous system involvement is a particular feature of some of these cases. Current approaches to prevent infectious complications focus on measures to accelerate and improve the quality of immunological recovery after immunosuppression; the use of colony stimulating factors as an adjunct to drug therapy of invasive aspergillosis, and active immunization.

REFERENCES

Barnes RA & Rogers TR (1987) An evaluation of empirical antibiotic therapy in febrile neutropenic patients. *British Journal of Haematology* **66:** 137–140.

Barnes RA & Rogers TR (1988) Response rates to a staged antibiotic regimen in febrile neutropenic patients. *Journal of Antimicrobial Chemotherapy* **22:** 137–140.

Barnes RA & Rogers TR (1989) Control of an outbreak of nosocomial aspergillosis by laminar airflow isolation. *Journal of Hospital Infection* **14:** 89–94.

Bodey GP, Anaissie E, Gutterman J & Vadhan-Raj S (1994) Role of granulocyte-macrophage colony-stimulating factor as adjuvant treatment in neutropenic patients with bacterial and fungal infection. *European Journal of Clinical Microbiology and Infectious Diseases* **13 (supplement 2):** 18–22.

Bowden RA & Meyers JD (1994) Infection complicating bone marrow transplantation. In Rubin RH & Young LS (eds) *Clinical Approach to Infection in the Compromised Host*, pp 601–628. New York: Plenum Medical.

Bowden RA, Sayers M, Gleaves CA et al (1987) Cytomegalovirus-seronegative blood components for the prevention of primary cytomegalovirus infection after marrow transplantation. *Transfusion* **27:** 478–481.

Brunell P, Shehab Z, Geiser C et al (1982) Administration of live varicella vaccine to children with leukaemia. *Lancet* ***ii:*** 1069–1072.

Centers for Disease Control (1984) Varicella-zoster immune globulin for the prevention of chickenpox: recommendations of the Immunization Practices Advisory Committee. *Annals of Internal Medicine* **100:** 859–865.

Chen PY, Chu HY, Shian WJ et al (1994) Varicella-zoster virus infection in children with malignancy. *Chung Hua I Hseuh Tsa Chih Taipei* **54:** 417–423.

Childers NK, Stinnett EA, Wheeler P et al (1993) Oral complications in children with cancer. *Oral Surgery Oral Medicine Oral Pathology* **75:** 41–47.

Cone RW, Hackman RC, Huang MW et al (1993) Human herpes virus in lung tissue from patients with pneumonitis after bone marrow transplantation. *New England Journal of Medicine* **329:** 156–161.

Cowie F, Meller ST, Cushing P & Pinkerton R (1994) Chemoprophylaxis for pulmonary aspergillosis during intensive chemotherapy. *Archives of Diseases in Childhood* **2:** 136–138.

Darbyshire PJ, Weightman WC & Speller DCE (1985) Problems associated with indwelling central venous catheters. *Archives of Disease in Childhood* **60:** 129–124.

Diaz PS, Au D, Smith S et al (1991) Lack of transmission of the live attenuated varicella vaccine virus to immunocompromised children after immunization of their siblings. *Pediatrics* **87:** 166–170.

Donnelly JP, Maschmeyer G & Daene S (1992) Selective oral antimicrobial prophylaxis for the prevention of infection in acute leukaemia—ciprofloxacin versus co-trimoxazole plus colistin. *European Journal of Cancer* **28A:** 878.

Fink FM, Hocker-Schulz S, Mor W et al (1993) Association of hepatitis C infection with chronic liver disease in paediatric cancer patients. *European Journal of Paediatrics* **152:** 490–492.

Foot AB, Oakhill A & Mott MG (1990) Cryptosporidiosis and acute leukaemia. *Archives of Diseases in Childhood* **65:** 236–237.

Gerson AA, Steinberg SP, Gelb L et al (1984) Live attenuated varicella vaccine: efficacy for children with leukemia in remission. *Journal of the American Medical Association* **255:** 355–362.

Gisselbrecht C, Prentice HG, Bacigalupo A et al (1994) Placebo-controlled phase III trial of lenograstim in bone-marrow transplantation. *Lancet* **343:** 696–700.

Hertz MI, Englund JA & Snover D et al (1989) Respiratory syncytial virus-induced acute lung injury in adult patients with bone marrow transplants: a clinical approach and review of the literature. *Medicine* **68:** 269–281.

Koch WC, Massey G, Russell CE et al (1990) Manifestations and treatment of human parvovirus B19 infection in immunocompromised patients. *Journal of Pediatrics* **116:** 355–359.

Kurtzman GJ, Cohen B, Meyers P et al (1988) Persistent B19 parvovirus infection as a cause of severe chronic anaemia in children with acute lymphocytic leukaemia. *Lancet* **ii:** 1159–1162.

Lawrence R, Gerson AA, Holzman R et al (1988) The risk of zoster after varicella vaccination in children with leukemia. *New England Journal of Medicine* **318:** 543–548.

Ljungman P, Cordonnier C, de Bock R et al (1995) Immunisations after bone marrow transplantation: results of a European survey and recommendations from the infectious diseases working party of the European group for Blood and Marrow Transplantation. *Bone Marrow Transplantation* **15:** 455–460.

Marina NM Flynn PM, Rivera GK & Hughes WT (1991) *Candida tropicalis* and *Candida albicans* fungemia in children with leukemia. *Cancer* **68:** 594–599.

Mirro JJr, Rao BN, Kumar M et al (1990) A comparison of placement techniques and complications of externalized catheters and implantable port use in children with cancer. *Journal of Pediatric Surgery* **25:** 120–124.

Moore L, Ellis DH, Suppiah R et al (1993) Complete eradication of *Aspergillus fumigatus* from the lung in an immunocompromised patient by oral itraconazole. *Journal of Paediatric Child Health* **29:** 141–143.

Pizzo PA, Robichaud RN, Wesley R & Commers JR (1982) Fever in the pediatric and young adult patient with cancer. *Medicine* **61:** 153–165.

Prentice A, Warnock DW, Johnson SAN et al (1994) Multiple dose pharmacokinetics of an oral solution of itraconozole in autologous bone marrow transplant recipients. *Journal of Antimicrobial Chemotherapy* **34:** 247–252.

Pullan C, Noble TC, Scott DJ, et al (1976) Atypical measles infections in leukaemic children on immunosuppressive treatment. *British Medical Journal* **i:** 1562–1565.

Rogers TR (1990) Infections associated with immunodeficiency In Parker MT & Collier LH (eds) *Principles of Bacteriology Virology and Immunity*, pp 173–196. London: Edward Arnold.

Rogers TR (1994) Fungal infections. In Burnett A (ed) *Haematological Oncology*, vol 3, pp 225–242. Cambridge: Cambridge University Press.

Rogers TR & Selwyn S (1994) Infections complicating bone marrow transplantation. In Jenkins GC & Williams JD (eds) *Infection and Haematology*, pp 183–200. Oxford: Butterworth-Heineman Press.

Rogers TR, Petrou MA, Lucas C et al (1981) Spread of *Clostridium difficile* among patients receiving non-absorbable antibiotics for gut decontamination. *British Medical Journal* **283:** 408–409.

Rogers TR, Riches PG, Walker SA & Joshi R (1986) Changes in immunoglobulin levels and implications for immunoglobulin therapy to prevent infection following bone marrow transplantation. In Morell A & Nydegger VE (eds) *Clinical Use of Intravenous Immunoglobulin*. London: Academic Press.

Rogers TR, Haynes KA & Barnes RA (1990) Value of antigen detection in predicting invasive pulmonary aspergillosis. *Lancet* **336:** 1210–1213.

Rokicka-Milewska R, Jackowsa T, Sopylo B & Seyfried H (1993) Active immunization of children with leukemias and lymphomas against infection by hepatitis B virus. *Acta Paediatrica Japan* **35:** 400–403.

Schmidt GM, Horak DA, Niland JC et al (1991) A randomized, controlled trial of prophylactic ganciclovir for cytomegalovirus pulmonary infection in recipients of allogeneic bone marrow transplant; The City of Hope-Stanford–Syntex CMV Study Group. *New England Journal of Medicine* **324:** 1005–1011.

Sheldon J, Riches PG, Soni N et al (1991) Plasma neopterin as an adjunct to C-reactive protein in assessment of infection. *Clinical Chemistry* **37:** 2038–2042.

Siegel MM Walter TK & Ablin AR (1977) Measles pneumonia in childhood leukemia. *Pediatrics* **60:** 38–40.

Takaue Y, Okamoto Y, Kawano Y et al (1994) Regeneration of immunity and varicella zoster virus infection after high-dose chemotherapy and peripheral blood stem cell autografts in children. *Bone Marrow Transplantation* **14:** 219–223.

Tang CM, Holden DW, Aufauvre-Brown A & Cohen J (1993) The detection of *Aspergillus* spp by the polymerase chain reaction and its evaluation in bronchoalveolar lavage fluid. *American Review of Respiratory Disease* **148:** 1313–1317.

Turner ML, Russell L, Milne & Parker AC (1993) Invasive aspergillosis in two patients with acute lymphoblastic leukaemia in complete remission. *Postgraduate Medical Journal* **69:** 405–408.

Uderzo C, D'Angelo P & Rizzari C et al (1992) Central venous catheter-related complications after bone marrow transplantation in children with haematological malignancies. *Bone Marrow Transplantation* **9:** 113–117.

Vossen JM, Heidt PJ, Van den Berg H et al (1990) Prevention of infection and graft-versus-host disease by suppression of intestinal microflora in children treated with allogeneic bone marrow transplantation. *European Journal of Clinical Microbiology and Infectious Diseases* **9:** 14–23.

Walker SA, Rogers TR, Riches PG et al (1984) Value of serum C-reactive protein measurement in the management of bone marrow transplant recipients. Part I: early transplant period. *Journal of Clinical Pathology* **37:** 1018–1021.

Wingard JR, Merz WG, Rinaldi MG et al (1991) Increase in *Candida krusei* infection among patients with bone marrow transplantation and neutropenia treated prophylactically with fluconazole. *New England Journal of Medicine* **325:** 1274–1277.

Young LS (1994) Management of infections in leukemia and lymphoma. In Rubin RH & Young LS (eds) *Clinical Approach to Infection in the Compromised Host*, pp 551–579. New York: Plenum Medical.

4

Psychosocial support and symptom management

ANN GOLDMAN

The diagnosis of leukaemia or lymphoma in a child has a profound impact on any family. This remains the case in spite of the overall improvement in prognosis and the increased emphasis on multidisciplinary and psychosocial support over recent years.

Treatment for leukaemia and lymphoma is complex and involves many aspects of care and many different professionals. This can easily lead to confusion and misunderstanding both for the families and between professionals. Treatment aimed at cure of the illness, symptom management and psychosocial support need to run alongside each other and be well integrated. During the changing course of the child's illness, different problems will become important. In response to this, different aspects of care will become more prominent. Since care for the majority of families is shared between the oncology referral centre, the local paediatric department and the primary health care team, good communication and coordination are essential.

SYMPTOM MANAGEMENT

It is essential to aim for high-quality symptom management throughout a child's illness. For the two-thirds of children who will be cured of leukaemia or lymphoma the suffering experienced from treatment and its side-effects will be what they remember. A recent study of long-term survivors has shown that subsequent stress was related to children's subjective appraisal of treatment intensity (Stuber et al, 1994). For those children who unfortunately cannot be cured, palliative care, including rigorous attention to symptom management, will help to provide as good a quality of life as possible for the time that remains.

During treatment

Procedures

It is easy for an adult to underestimate the fear and pain experienced by many children for what seem relatively small procedures, such as finger

Baillière's Clinical Paediatrics—
Vol. 3, No. 4, November 1995
ISBN 0–7020–2075–3

pricks and insertion of peripheral intravenous lines. Providing help for these procedures as early as possible is important in order to try to prevent anxiety and subsequent problems. Careful and honest preparation of the child and parents can be combined with the use of a local anaesthetic cream (Clarke and Radford, 1986) and age appropriate distraction techniques (Kuttner, 1989). Action for Sick Children have a helpful leaflet for parents 'Needles—helping to take away the fear' (Action for Sick Children, 1994). Indwelling central catheters avoid the problems of repeated invasive access and are used increasingly. However, they have complications and may not be appropriate for all children.

More invasive procedures, such as bone marrow aspirates and lumbar punctures, can cause considerable distress. Although some older children will tolerate these with local anaesthetic, sometimes augmented by distraction and hypnosis (Zeltzer and LeBaron, 1982), sedation with analgesia or general anaesthesia are usually used. Approaches at different centres vary and include the use of ketamine, midazolam, nitrous oxide and fentanyl (Anderson et al, 1993). Early preparation of the children and parents and co-ordinating a number of procedures at the same time helps to minimize distress.

Nausea and vomiting

Nausea and vomiting are among the most distressing side-effects of chemotherapy. They cause misery to the children, upset to the parents and can, in extreme cases, lead to treatment refusal. Managing nausea and vomiting aggressively from the start helps to gain the confidence of the child and parents, and reduces the difficult problem of anticipatory vomiting.

The emetogenic potential of chemotherapy agents varies (Table 1). They may exert their effects both centrally, through the chemoreceptor trigger zone and peripherally, through the gastro intestinal tract. Children also vary in their susceptibility, with anticipatory vomiting more common in older children and adolescents.

A variety of anti-emetics are available and have been used over the years in varying doses, both alone and in combination (Table 2). The vast majority of drug trials have been in adults. Satisfactory studies have been difficult to design because of the large number of variables which need to be co-ordinated. Undoubtedly the greatest advance has been the introduction of the 5-HT antagonists (Pinkerton et al, 1990). These drugs offer a considerable improvement in anti-emesis and are now used routinely for the more intensely emetogenic protocols. However, they are more expensive and this has resulted in some reluctance to introduce them for protocols which are only moderately emetogenic. Others have suggested that when the overall costs of using cheaper but less effective drugs are calculated, the difference is relatively small (Cunningham et al, 1993).

Different oncology centres vary in their preferences and approach. For drugs with very low emetogenic incidence no anti-emetic is required. With those which are highly emetogenic a 5-HT antagonist would be a first

Table 1. Emetogenic potential of some chemotherapy agents.

High
Cisplatin
Cyclophosphamide
Ifosfamide
Melphelan
Moderate
Actinomycin
Amsacrine
Asparaginase
Carboplatin
Chlorambucil
Cytarabine
Daunorubicin
Doxorubicin
Methotrexate (high-dose)
Procarbazine
Low
Bleomycin
Etoposide
Methotrexate (low-dose)
Vincristine

Table 2. Anti-emetics and their sites of action.

Anti-emetic	Site of action
Anticholinergics	
hyoscine	Vomiting centre
Antihistamines	
cyclizine	Vomiting centre
Dopamine antagonists	
phenothiazines	Ctz
butyrephenones	Ctz
metoclopramide	Ctz, periphery
domperidone	Ctz, periphery
$5HT^3$ antagonists	Ctz, periphery
Steroids	Unknown

Ctz = chemoreceptor trigger zone.

choice and, if vomiting persists, this can be augmented with dexamethasone. More variation occurs for the intermediate chemotherapy agents and the child's individual preference and susceptibility must also be considered. Phenothiazines or metaclopramide may relieve emesis sufficiently and are cheaper. Unfortunately they are often inadequate and are more likely to cause side-effects. A 5-HT antagonist will then need to be introduced, and in the meantime the child will have suffered and lost confidence.

Since most chemotherapeutic agents require intravenous access, anti-emetics can also be given, initially, via the same route. If the child is an in-patient, the anti-emetic can be given some time before the chemotherapy so that an effective blood level has been established. In out-patients, anti-emetics can be given intravenously just prior to the chemotherapy, or parents can give an oral dose at home in anticipation. It is important to provide oral or rectal drugs for the child to continue to use when they return home.

Pain

Pain may arise from the effects of the tumour itself at diagnosis. This may include bone pain from marrow engorgement, abdominal pain from liver and splenic enlargement and headache from CNS involvement. The most effective treatment will be the chemotherapy directed at the disease, which usually leads to rapid relief. However, it may be necessary to provide analgesics to cover the period of investigation and until the disease remits. Drugs can be chosen in the same way as for a child with progressive disease (see below).

Mucositis with severe pain is frequently experienced by children having high-dose chemotherapy or total body irradiation with bone marrow transplantation. As well as local mouth care strong opioid drugs are often required, which will need to be given by continuous infusion as the child will not be able to take oral preparation. In older children, patient-controlled analgesia can be considered, although a baseline analgesic infusion is usually needed as well as patient-controlled boosts (Lloyd-Thomas, 1990).

The dying child

Pain

A great fear for parents who know their child is dying is that he or she will suffer pain. This is a realistic concern as we found that 87% of children dying from progressive malignant disease required strong opioid analgesics. Although a number (17%) needed them for less than 24 hours, 70% required them for longer (Goldman et al, 1990). The nature of the pain will depend on the sites and spread of the disease. The pain should be assessed to distinguish the different sites, the nature and the cause of the pain so that appropriate treatment can be chosen. It is possible to provide good pain relief for the majority of children, although there are some for whom it is not complete; neuropathic pain in particular can be a problem.

Assessment of pain in children can be difficult because of their limited understanding and communication skills. Clinicians tend to rely on history from the parents and clinical examination, but a range of specific pain assessment tools for children have been developed in recent years. The majority of these depend on subjective assessment by the child and can be chosen according to their age and ability. Body charts are helpful for all ages to locate and identify sites of pain, while colour scales, faces, numeric and visual analogue scales can be used to measure severity (Mathews et al,

1993). Formal assessment can be particularly helpful when judging the value of different treatment regimens.

Since pain is a complex sensation influenced by psychological, social and cultural factors as well as the physical damage to the tissues it is often helpful to combine a variety of different approaches in its treatment (Table 3).

Table 3. Approaches to pain management.

Analgesics
non-opioid
mild opioid
strong opioid
amitriptyline, anticonvulsants
Anticancer therapy
radiotherapy
chemotherapy
Anaesthetic
EMLA
sedation or inhalation
regional blocks
Psychological
educational, explanation
distraction
relaxation
hypnosis
Physical
warmth, cold
massage, physiotherapy
TENS

Analgesics of increasing strength can be introduced, in accordance with the World Health Organisation's concept of an analgesic ladder (World Health Organisation, 1986). Paracetamol is the mild non-opioid drug usually chosen in children. It acts peripherally, is helpful in mild to moderate pain and has few side-effects. When pain relief is no longer achieved by regular paracetamol a mild opioid such as dihydrocodeine can be introduced. Potential side-effects are similar to morphine (see below). In practice the important problem to anticipate is constipation, and laxatives should be prescribed routinely. The analgesic effect of codeine also has a ceiling and when it no longer relieves the pain a strong opioid is needed.

Morphine sulphate is the oral opioid used most commonly. It is essential to give it regularly; 4-hourly or 12-hourly, slow-release preparations are available. The slow-release preparations are especially convenient for care in the child's home, but a short-acting morphine sulphate preparation must also always be provided, to use for breakthrough pain (Goldman and Bowman, 1990). Starting doses can be estimated according to the child's weight, and regular re-assessment is required so that the dose is increased to provide optimum analgesia.

Oral analgesics in increasing doses provide adequate analgesia for most children until their death. Sometimes, as the child becomes more poorly, drugs can no longer be taken orally and an alternative route is needed. Rectal medication can be considered and some children tolerate this well, preferring it to the thought of any needles. It is also often appropriate when the child is no longer conscious or for the last few hours. Morphine suppositories are available and MST tablets (in the same dose as orally) can be used rectally (Wilkinson et al, 1992). Drugs can also conveniently be given, at home, by continuous infusion using a simple pump. Usually the needle is subcutaneous but if a central indwelling intravenous catheter is in situ this can also be used. Diamorphine is usually substituted for morphine because of its greater solubility.

Strong opioids have many side-effects. The main one causing clinical problems is constipation. Laxatives should always be prescribed prophylactically. Drowsiness is also common at first but this almost always wears off within 2 or 3 days. It is useful to warn parents that their child is likely to become drowsy or they may worry that the disease has suddenly progressed. Nausea and vomiting are uncommon and so anti-emetics are not necessary prophylactically. Some children experience itching; this usually also wears off but, if not, antihistamines are helpful.

Professionals who rarely use opioid drugs in children may be concerned about potential respiratory depression, but there appears to be a wide margin between the dose causing respiratory failure and that required for analgesia. Pain has been described as a physiological antagonist to the respiratory depressant effects of morphine (Hanks and Twycross, 1984).

Sometimes parents are reluctant to consider the use of morphine for their child's pain. In order to overcome this the reasons for their concern need to be explored. Often it is not the use of morphine itself but that it represents an acknowledgement that the child is actually dying. They may also be confused about addiction and need reassurance that psychological addiction does not seem to occur in children requiring opioids for cancer pain. In addition, although tolerance will develop, should the pain be relieved (for example by radiotherapy) then the morphine dose can easily be tapered and then stopped.

Although it is well known that non-steroidal anti-inflammatory drugs are helpful in bone pain in cancer, they are not usually recommended for children with leukaemia and lymphoma as their platelet counts are already likely to be low. Nerve pain is uncommon in children with leukaemias and lymphomas but, if present, it may be helped by carbamazepine or low-dose amitriptyline. Headaches from central nervous system disease are most effectively relieved by intrathecal chemotherapy.

Anaemia and thrombocytopenia

The majority of children with progressive leukaemia and lymphoma become anaemic during the course of their terminal illness. There may be a dilemma as to whether or not it is appropriate to transfuse them or not. Regular monitoring of blood counts and platelet counts is not necessary during palliative care as treatment is offered in response to symptoms. If the child has enjoyed a good quality of life until the onset of the symptoms from anaemia then transfusion is often helpful and appropriate. Eventually, as the child becomes more ill, the benefits of transfusion diminish and a time is reached when transfusion is no longer appropriate. If this has been discussed from the outset with the parents then the decision to stop transfusions can be made mutually. Although many of the children have low platelets, in practice serious bleeding is uncommon. Platelet transfusions should be reserved for bleeding which interferes with the quality of life, for example, nose bleeds or haematemesis, but not just for petechiae. Children who have had a history of bleeding during their illness, or with promyelocytic leukaemia, may require more regular transfusions.

Other symptoms

Other symptoms which may need consideration are nausea and vomiting. Oral or rectal anti-emetics may be successful but if not cyclizine or haloperidol are both compatible with diamorphine and can be given subcutaneously by continuous infusion. Cyclizine is particularly helpful for the vomiting associated with central nervous system disease. Convulsions associated with central nervous system disease are not common but may occur. Families at home may be reassured by having rectal diazepam available. Recurrent convulsions not helped by rectal diazepam at the time, and oral anticonvulsants, can be managed at home with subcutaneous midazolam.

SUPPORT OF FAMILIES

The considerable literature relating to psychosocial support for children with malignant disease and their families has evolved alongside the improving clinical outcome (Van Dongen-Melman and Sanders-Woudstra, 1986; Cincotta, 1993). The focus has shifted gradually from identifying and addressing the problems associated with probable death to assessing those of living with a serious illness and an uncertain outcome. More recently, emphasis has been on the exploration of families' coping skills, the psychological impact of the cancer on long-term survivors and the best ways to provide psychosocial support.

Problems for families

At diagnosis

The time of diagnosis is one of turmoil for the family. Common initial reactions shared by the child and parents can include shock, disbelief, distress, anxiety, anger and guilt. If the child has been ill for some time, with a delayed and difficult diagnosis, there may be anger with staff but also a sense of relief. Past priorities and patterns of life for the family are disrupted, many practical difficulties arise in day to day living, and it is easy for the parents and child to feel overwhelmed, helpless and out of control. There are difficulties because of the separation of the parents from each other, from their other children and from their community support network. There may be concerns about travel, time off work and finance, and all of these are superimposed on the grief of the diagnosis.

The child himself faces the trauma of being in hospital and the experience of unpleasant and frightening investigations and treatment. He is often particularly confused as explanations and understanding of what is happening may be delayed. Parents are themselves just learning about the illness and its treatment and may find discussing it with the child almost impossible.

During treatment

During treatment the child and family continue to experience stress. They live with the underlying conflict of maintaining hope in spite of persistent uncertainty. Parents may develop depression, anxiety and sleep disturbance although they are often reluctant to speak of these problems unless asked specifically. Marital discord and loss of libido are also widely reported. Practical problems of travel, separation and finance continue. Parents often find new difficulties in handling the children, particularly in maintaining discipline and boundaries for the sick child and also balancing their time and emotions between the sick child and well siblings. Around the time that treatment is completed can be an anxious period for parents, as their fears of relapse re-emerge, without the reassurance of regular chemotherapy.

The sick child continues to experience regular hospital visits, the intensive treatment and unpleasant side-effects. His understanding of the illness and the therapy develop alongside the experience. His life at home is disrupted and gradually family relationships, friendships, school and activities must all be re-established, in the light of the illness.

Long-term survivors

Since the majority of children are now cured of cancer, defining the long-term physical and psychological sequelae has become increasingly important. This is addressed comprehensively in Chapter 8. Although definite long-term psychological problems are acknowledged (Pi Nian Chang, 1991) it is also encouraging that survivors are also able to recognise positive effects of their experience. Many feel more mature than their peers and identify a more positive outlook and sense of purpose in their lives (Lozowski, 1993).

After relapse

If a child relapses, the family is forced to face the life-threatening nature of the illness again, even more clearly than at diagnosis. The emotional impact of relapse can be particularly dramatic for parents who have held a very positive and 'fighting' approach throughout treatment. For others it is a confirmation of what they have dreaded and felt was inevitable all along. The shock felt at diagnosis and all the emotions accompanying it may re-emerge.

At this time the oncologist and family must make choices about future treatment; whether it is possible to aim for a cure, whether the side-effects of further aggressive therapy are balanced by the likelihood of a good remission or whether the time has come to focus on palliative care only. Whatever the decision, this is a time of crisis for the child and the family, who will need answers to their questions and time to discuss their fears and feelings.

Even if further treatment against the tumour is instituted, for most children who relapse there comes a time when medical staff believe that cure is no longer possible. Although discussing this with a family and acknowledging that death is inevitable can be very difficult, it offers an opportunity to confront the situation openly. The stress of uncertainty is removed and problems can be anticipated and planned for.

Providing help

Families whose children develop cancer are ordinary people, experiencing an extreme psychological trauma in their lives. Support and care needs to focus on ways to help them cope with this, while enabling them to continue to function and develop as normally as possible throughout the illness and into the future. A balance must be sought in which the child and family's problems are acknowledged, without over-emphasizing them and so disabling and damaging the family's own inner resources (Chesler, 1993).

All families need empathy and sensitivity in their care from all members of the team. Formal explicit psychological support should also be available to all families, from staff with appropriate training. This is usually provided by specialist social workers or psychologists, though experienced nurses, play specialists, chaplains and doctors may take this role at different times and for different members of the family. Paediatric oncology community nurse specialists have the valuable opportunity of working with families in their own homes (Cribb et al, 1994). Unique support comes from other parents, either informally or through organized groups. They realise they are not alone in their fears, and can learn from the experience of others.

Families at risk

In spite of the many studies demonstrating emotional distress, the majority of families do possess considerable strength and resilience and find a way to continue to function effectively from day to day. A number of factors have been identified which can help to predict a family's capacity to cope, although formal family assessment tools are not used routinely.

Cohesive, supportive, flexible families do better than over-involved or unconnected and rigid ones. A pattern of open communication within the family and with the medical and nursing team is one of the most positive predictors of coping. Concurrent stress in the family, previous parental psychopathology and a poor record of coping with past stresses suggests an increased risk of problems (Kupst, 1993).

Coping strategies

Van Dongen-Melman, after an extensive review of the literature (Van Dongen-Melman and Sanders-Woudstra 1986), suggests that families coping with childhood cancer develop strategies in order to reduce uncertainty, gain and maintain control of the situation, maintain and protect self esteem and to reduce negative feelings (Van Dongen-Melman et al, 1986).

One of the important strategies families employ to reduce uncertainty and gain some sense of control is to seek information. This may be through formal sources such as hospital staff, or books, or informally through friends and other families with cancer. Accurate information is a powerful method of reducing uncertainty. Children, both the sick child and the siblings, also need to find out what is happening. This includes both knowledge about the illness itself and also about treatment and procedures. Without appropriate information they turn to their imagination or to informal, and sometimes unreliable, sources. Horrifying fantasies, inappropriate self blame and guilt may develop. Both for children and adults the fear of the unknown is worse than the reality (Bluebond-Langner, 1978).

Expressing feelings, especially negative ones, openly and receiving reassurance and support can be helpful. Patients and families who are able to do this together have fewer problems. However, many families also value the opportunity to talk to someone less close, and other families, friends, social workers and medical staff can provide this. Some families choose to avoid all discussion and may appear to deny the seriousness of the illness entirely. This should be explored; an extreme position is unusual and unhelpful and may require professional intervention. However, most families employ some avoidance and denial as part of their coping strategy and this is normal. It can protect them from extremes of emotion and allow them to understand and recognise the situation gradually. Some use of denial allows the child and family to live with the illness and function normally.

The most active coping strategy is to try and change the situation. Discussing treatment protocols, beginning therapy and becoming involved in nursing and medical tasks is part of this. It is valuable for the family to be involved and feel that they are members of the team, actively working towards improving the situation. Families wish to take on different levels of responsibility and care, and staff must remain sensitive and flexible. Planning towards the return to school and developing appropriate goals for the future are other active approaches to coping. Even when it is no longer possible to offer a cure, the family can continue to work with the team towards a peaceful death.

Professionals working with families can help them to identify their immediate problems, and clarify and express their feelings. Every family and individual within a family is different and will have their own personal strengths and coping mechanisms. If professionals can recognise this, in a non-judgmental way, they can work with them both as individuals and as a family.

The dying child

Even though stopping treatment against the tumour is a difficult decision, usually it is one that can be made mutually, with the family. Some families will be helped by the offer of a second opinion. A few will continue to search, aggressively, for a cure until the child's death.

At this terrible time it is important to stress to the family that physical care and support for the sick child and themselves will continue, so that they do not feel abandoned. Staff need to respond to each family individually. Some families want to talk through the situation in great detail immediately and want as much information as possible, others prefer to build up a picture gradually, as the child's condition changes.

It is essential to address practical aspects of care and to discuss whether the family wants to be at home, who is available to help them, what the likely symptoms may be and how they can be tackled. What to say to the sick child, brothers and sisters, and to the wider family, is often a major concern for parents. Other questions may be unspoken, but cause great fear and distress—what happens at the moment of death, how can we be planning a funeral while she is still alive, is it terrible to wish it was all over? Each family needs someone from the oncology team with the skill, confidence and time to help them consider all these questions and the multitude of feelings they invoke.

Communicating with children

Anxiety is commonly reduced in children, just as it is in adults, when they understand and can anticipate events (Kendrick et al, 1987). The consensus in the literature is that children understand and learn about their illness and its implications, whether their parents and the professionals encourage it or not. It also appears that the children benefit from being encouraged to discuss their questions and concerns openly (Bluebond-Langner, 1978; Spinetta and Deasy-Spinetta, 1981).

Although staff favour openness in discussion with children it can be difficult in practice, particularly when a child has relapsed and death is a real possibility. Even experienced oncology staff routinely use distancing tactics when working with cancer patients (Maguire, 1985). Many children rely mainly on their parents for information, and the few studies looking at discussion within families, at diagnosis (Chesler et al, 1986) and during terminal care (Goldman and Christie 1993), suggest that it remains an area where families need considerable help and support.

Communication with children must take into consideration their level of understanding about illness (Eiser, 1985) and death (Lansdown and Benjamin, 1985). It will also be influenced by the child's experience, their family's style of communication and their own personal defence mechanisms. It need not rely only on talking, and children are particularly good at sensing non-verbal messages. Drawing, stories and play are often easier and more effective ways to explain to children what is happening and for them to express their fears and emotions.

The child at school

School is a regular part of the life of all children. Encouraging and facilitating children with malignant disease to continue to attend school as much as possible is important and is much preferred to establishing home tuition. As well as providing essential continuing education, it represents normality, offers them a respite from being different and the opportunity to maintain relationships and activities with their peers.

A variety of difficulties relating to school have been identified for children with cancer. These include problems with re-entry, frequent periods of absence, physical problems related to treatment, changes in behaviour and mood, and higher rates of learning difficulties (Deasy-Spinetta, 1981; Larcombe et al, 1990). Clearly, children vary, and each one's problems must be assessed individually.

Teachers have also identified the dilemmas that they face when children return to school. They report a conflict in obtaining information while respecting a family's privacy. They also found it difficult to know what were appropriate academic expectations, what medical problems to expect, and how to determine appropriate levels of discipline and emotional support. They also identified the personal impact they felt of having a child with cancer in their class (Deasy-Spinetta, 1981; Chekryn et al, 1987).

Identification of these problems has highlighted the need for the hospital to help both in re-integrating the child into school and in identifying children's cognitive and academic difficulties. In the past, parents have often been left to provide schools with information. Additional direct liaison by a member of the hospital team with the school can provide more effective information and support for staff. It offers school staff the opportunity to discuss both the physical and psychological problems openly, without fear of distressing the parents. Many paediatric oncology community nurse specialists now regularly make school visits (Hunt, 1994). Other initiatives include inviting teachers of newly diagnosed children to study days at the hospital and the provision of specific literature for schools (Larcombe).

Children with problems, or those particularly at risk, such as those who have had cranial irradiation, should be formally assessed. Thereafter, in the UK, a local education authority 'has an obligation to make appropriate arrangements to meet them and keep them under review' (Education Act 1981). Unfortunately, in practice, levels of support can vary considerably.

The bereaved family

Grief is the normal response to death, but the grief suffered after the loss of a child is described as the most painful, enduring and difficult to survive (Hindmarch, 1993) and it is associated with a high risk of pathological grief. Parents lose not only the child they have loved but their hopes for the future and confidence in themselves as parents. Siblings suffer the loss of their brother or sister. In addition, they often feel isolated and neglected as their parents can spare little energy and emotion for them. Many siblings have behavioural problems and difficulty adjusting (Pettle-Michael and Lansdown, 1986).

Families of children dying from leukaemia and lymphoma have often developed close relationships with hospital staff. Offering support to them through their bereavement is an extension of the care for the family during the illness. Hospitals vary in how much they are able to provide. Some families do not welcome continued contact, so individual arrangements should be planned. Paediatric oncology clinical nurse specialists or social workers will often be able to provide a period of intensive and then gradually decreasing support to parents and siblings. Ideally, this should involve facilitating the normal tasks of mourning and expressions of grief (Worden, 1991). They can provide information about appropriate literature, telephone helplines and groups. It is also important for staff to be able to recognise when there are signs of pathology which require them to initiate specialist bereavement counselling. Even if resources do not allow home visits, most families appreciate members of the hospital staff attending funerals, sending flowers, and cards or telephone contact made on birthdays or anniversaries of the child's death. This offers a continuing link and the chance for families to ask if they feel they need more help.

SHARED CARE

With local hospitals

The majority of children with leukaemia and lymphoma are treated under the supervision of paediatric oncology centres. It has been demonstrated that the outcome for these children is significantly improved compared to those treated elsewhere (Stiller, 1988). Over the years many centres have developed a system of shared care with local paediatric centres. This enables the centre to make optimal use of its expertise and specialist facilities and has the advantage, for the family, of reducing travel and disruption. It is also a philosophy which many local paediatricians value (Bacon, 1989).

The UK Childrens Cancer Study Group (UKCCSG) centres vary considerably in the extent to which they practice shared care and how they arrange to do it. There has been remarkably little formal assessment of the process. One study (Muir et al, 1992) has demonstrated that the prognosis in ALL is not compromised when shared care is offered to patients identified as suitable by the oncologist. However, the other benefits and disadvantages to the child and families, the standards needed by the participating hospitals and the best ways of communicating and providing care are still unclear.

Bacon (1989) states that 'a good relationship between peripheral and regional paediatricians has to be worked at. It requires mutual respect and courtesy . . .'. This type of relationship must also extend to local and regional nursing staff, junior medical staff and all those involved in care for the families to benefit fully. Communication between centres can be enhanced by a variety of approaches. Regionally based paediatric oncology community nurse specialists can visit district hospitals and make personal contact with local staff. They act as a visible link for families and can also provide teaching and support locally. Patient-held notes, which families carry with them between various centres, provide a personalized and up-to-date record (Hully and Hyne, 1993). Multidisciplinary study days at the regional centre offer an opportunity for formal teaching and also for staff to get to know each other informally.

With the community

The family doctor and primary health care team can sometimes find themselves excluded when a child and family are spending a lot of time receiving hospital care. The family rapidly become expert in their child's illness, and the community staff can feel uncomfortable and de-skilled. However, throughout treatment, and particularly for those children who are not going to be cured, a supportive and involved primary health care team is very valuable. The hospital can encourage their involvement through regular communication, and by providing up-to-date information about the child's illness and treatment. Some centres provide written information packs at the time of diagnosis (James et al, 1988). Paediatric oncology nurse specialists can also visit practices and discuss individual children and their care.

SUMMARY

Psychosocial support and symptom management are important from the time of diagnosis, and need to run alongside treatment aiming to cure the disease. During treatment, fear and pain from procedures should be anticipated. Preparatory explanations, play and distraction should be augmented with the use of local anaesthetic creams and sedation or anaesthesia for more invasive procedures. Nausea and vomiting from chemotherapy should be treated aggressively. For children with progressive and terminal disease pain is an important problem and influenced by psychological, social and cultural factors as well as tissue damage. Analgesics of increasing strength can be combined with psychological and other approaches to relieve pain. The role of blood and platelet transfusion and management of other symptoms is also considered. Support for families throughout treatment must balance acknowledging their problems and offering help without disabling and damaging their own inner resources. Professionals can help the sick child and members of the family identify problems, clarify and express their feelings, and recognize and enhance their coping skills. Children benefit from an open style of communication within the family and also between the family and professionals. Children should be encouraged to attend school and this can be facilitated by direct contact with teachers. Bereaved families can be supported through the normal tasks of mourning and those requiring specialist counselling identified. Co-operation between paediatric oncology centres, local hospitals and primary health care teams is essential and some ways of facilitating this are suggested.

REFERENCES

Action for Sick Children (1994) Family Information series 1994 *Needles—helping to take away the fear*. Available from Action for Sick Children, 29–31, Euston Road, London NW1 2SD. Tel. 0171.833.2041.

Anderson CTM, Zeltzer LK & Fanurik D (1993) Procedural pain. In Schechter NL, Berde CB and Yaster M (eds) *Pain in Infants, Children and Adolescents*, pp 435–458. Baltimore: Williams & Wilkins.

Bacon CJ (1989) Shared care in paediatrics. *Archives of Diseases in Childhood* **64:** 148–149.

Bluebond-Langner M (1978) *The Private Worlds of Dying Children*. Princeton, New Jersey: Princeton University Press.

Chekryn J, Deegan M & Reid J (1987) Impact on teachers when a child with cancer returns to school. *Children's Health Care* **15:** 161–165.

Chesler MA (1993) Introduction to psycho-social issues. *Cancer* **71 (supplement):** 3245–3250.

Chesler MA, Paris J & Barbarin OA (1986) 'Telling' the child with cancer: parental choices to share information with their children. *Journal of Paediatric Psychology* **11:** 497–515.

Cincotta N (1993) Psycho-social issues in the world of children with cancer. *Cancer* **71 (supplement):** 3251–3260.

Clarke S & Radford M (1986) Topical anaesthesia for venepuncture. *Archives of Disease of Childhood* **61:** 1132–1134.

Cribb A, Bignold S & Ball SJ (1994) Linking the parts: an exemplar of philosophical and practical issues in holistic nursing. *Journal of Advanced Nursing* **20:** 233–238.

Cunningham D, Gore M, Davidson N et al (1993) The real cost of emesis—an economic analysis of ondansetron vs metacloproamide in controlling emesis in patients receiving chemotherapy for cancer. *European Journal of Cancer* **29A:** 303–306.

Deasy-Spinetta P (1981) The school and the child with cancer. In Spinetta JJ and Deasy-Spinetta P (eds) *Living with Childhood Cancer*, pp 153–168. St Louis: CV Mosby.

Eiser C (1985) Changes in understanding of illness as the child grows. *Archives of Disease in Childhood* **60:** 489–492.

Goldman A & Bowman A (1990) The role of oral controlled release morphine for pain relief in children with cancer. *Palliative Medicine* **4:** 279–285.

Goldman & Christie D (1993) Children with cancer talk about their own death with their families. *Paediatric Haematology and Oncology* **10:** 223–231.

Goldman A, Beardsmore S & Hunt J (1990) Palliative care for children with cancer—home, hospital or hospice. *Archives of Diseases of Childhood* **65:** 641–643.

Hanks GW & Twycross RG (1984) Pain, the physiological antagonist of opioid analgesics. *Lancet* **i:** 1477–1478.

Hindmarch C (1993) *On the Death of A Child*. Oxford: Radcliffe Medical Press.

Hully M & Hyne J (1993) Using parent-held records in an oncology unit. *Paediatric Nursing* **5:** 14–16.

Hunt J (1994) Paediatric oncology clinical nurse specialists—towards a model of good practice. Interim report. Royal College of Nursing, London.

James JA, Harris DJ, Mott MG & Oakhill A (1988) Paediatric oncology information pack for general practitioners. *British Medical Journal* **296:** 97–98.

Kendrick C, Culling J, Oakhill T & Mott M (1987) Children's understanding of their illness and its treatment within a paediatric oncology unit. *Association of Child Psychology and Psychiatry* **8:** 16–25.

Kupst MJ (1993) Family coping: supportive and obstructive factors. *Cancer* **71 (supplement):** 3337–3341.

Kuttner L (1989) Management of young children's acute pain and anxiety during invasive procedures. *Paediatrician* **16:** 39–44.

Lansdown R & Benjamin G (1985) The development of the concept of death in children aged 5–9 years. *Child: Care, Health and Development* **11:** 13–20.

Larcombe IJ. *Welcome Back.* Available from Cancer Research Campaign Education and Child Studies Research Group, Department of Public Health and Epidemiology, Stopford Building, University of Manchester, Oxford Road, Manchester M13 9PT, UK.

Larcombe IJ, Walker J, Charlton A et al (1990) Impact of childhood cancer on return to normal schooling. *British Medical Journal* **301:** 169–171.

Lloyd Thomas AR (1990) Pain management in paediatric patients. *British Journal of Anaesthesia* **64:** 85–104.

Lozowski SL (1993) Views of childhood cancer survivors. *Cancer* **71 (supplement):** 3354–3357.

Maguire P (1985) Barriers to psychological care of the dying. *British Medical Journal* : 1711–1713.

Mathews JR, McGrath PJ & Pigeon H (1993) Assessment and measurement of pain in children. In Schechter NL, Berde CB and Yaster M (eds) *Pain in Infants, Children and Adolescents*, pp 97–111. Baltimore: Williams and Wilkins.

Muir KR, Parkes SE, Boon R et al (1992) Shared care in paediatric oncology. *Journal of Cancer Care* **1:** 15–17.

Pettle-Michael S & Lansdown R (1986) Adjustment to the death of a sibling. *Archives of Diseases in Childhood* **61:** 278–283.

Pi Nian Chang (1991) Psychosocial needs of long term childhood cancer survivors: a review of the literature. *Pediatrician* **18:** 20–24.

Pinkerton RC, Williams D, Wootton C et al (1990) 5-HT}3{ antagonist ondansetron—an effective outpatient antiemetic in cancer treatment. *Archives of Disease in Childhood* **65:** 822–825.

Spinetta JJ & Deasy-Spinetta P (1981) Talking with children who have a life threatening illness. In Spinetta JJ and Deasy-Spinetta P (eds) *Living with Childhood Cancer*, pp 234–252. St Louis: CV Mosby.

Stiller CA (1988) Centralisation of treatment and survival rates for cancer. *Archives of Disease in Childhood* **63:** 23–30.

Stuber ML, Meeske K, Gonzalez S et al (1994) Post traumatic stress after childhood cancer. 1: The role of appraisal. *Psycho-Oncology 3:* 305–312.

Van Dongen-Melman JEWM & Sanders-Woudstra JAR (1986) Psychosocial aspects of childhood cancer: a review of the literature. *Journal of Child Psychology and Psychiatry* **27:** 145–180.

Van Dongen-Melman JEWM, Pruyn JF, Van Zanen GE & Sanders-Woudstra JAR (1986) Coping with childhood cancer: a conceptual view. *Journal of Psychosocial Oncology* **4:** 147–161.

Wilkinson TJ, Robinson BA, Begg EJ et al (1992) Pharmacokinetics and efficacy of rectal versus oral sustained release morphine in cancer patients. *Cancer Chemotherapy and Pharmacology* **31:** 251–254.

Worden JW (1991) *Grief Counselling and Grief Therapy*, 2nd edn. London: Tavistock/Routledge.

World Health Organisation (1986) Cancer pain relief. Geneva.

Zeltzer L & LeBaron S (1982) Hypnosis and non-hypnotic techniques for reduction of pain and anxiety during painful procedures in children and adolescents with cancer. *Behavioural Pediatrics* **101:** 1032–1035.

5

Late effects following treatment of childhood leukaemia and lymphoma

MERIEL E. M. JENNEY
GEORGE D. N. KISSEN

The treatment of childhood leukaemia and lymphoma has become increasingly successful over the past 20 years. As a result, physical, psychological and social long-term effects of therapy are becoming more apparent. Some effects can be predicted (e.g. infertility following certain chemotherapeutic agents or gonadal irradiation); others are less well defined. This chapter summarizes those adverse sequelae known to occur in children treated for leukaemia and lymphoma. There is an emphasis on the effects of the treatment for leukaemia as they comprise the majority of surviving patients and have been most closely studied.

Identification of the late effects of treatment is important as intervention may be required (e.g. growth hormone replacement, psychological support) and delay may lead to further complications for the child. There are also wider implications, as future treatment protocols are planned, adverse effects of therapy may be minimized by modifications of treatment strategies. It is also important that the survivors themselves understand the issues they face and the implications any late effects have on their health. Clearly, however, the aim of therapy, that of cure, must not be forgotten or compromised.

The limitations of many of the studies of the late effects of therapy should be emphasized. The majority are cross-sectional and relate to a number of children treated at different times, often in different ways. The studies generally reflect the therapeutic trials of the past two decades, and it is of some concern that as the intensity of treatment increases (with improvements in survival), additional long-term complications will be seen. The value of the available data is to bring to light the problems many of the survivors face presently, which then may be anticipated and treated early. Prospective studies of whole cohorts of children with leukaemia and lymphoma are urgently required in order to define truly the extent of any late effects of treatment.

Historical perspective

As the treatment for leukaemia and lymphoma has evolved, so the pattern of late effects, which is largely related to the treatment received, has changed.

Baillière's Clinical Paediatrics—
Vol. 3, No. 4, November 1995
ISBN 0-7020-2075-3

However, the full effect of any changes will be apparent only years later. As cure rates rise so the emphasis on the control of late effects increases.

The treatment of ALL might be seen to be well advanced in this process. Initial success in the early 1960s (with regimens such as those developed at St Judes Children's Research Hospital, Memphis) was tempered by an unacceptably high rate of central nervous system (CNS) relapse (between 50 and 80%). The introduction of CNS-directed therapy in the form of craniospinal irradiation (St Judes Total Therapy for Childhood ALL Study VI, 1969) dramatically reduced CNS relapse rates and appeared to improve overall event-free survival. With time, the therapy was seen to have an effect on growth and educational achievement (Probert et al, 1973). The Medical Research Council UK ALL trials progressively reflected awareness of these sequelae. A step-wise change to cranial irradiation only (UKALL II, 1972: UKALL III, 1973), to avoid the myelosuppression of spinal irradiation and impairment of spinal growth, reduced dose cranial irradiation (UKALL VIII, 1980–4), and no cranial irradiation but alternative CNS-directed therapy for lower-risk (for CNS disease) patients (UKALL XI, 1991) has taken place as the late effects of each alternative strategy have been documented.

Alongside these changes the chemotherapeutic regimens have become progressively more intensive as improved cure and survival rates are seen. Cyclophosphamide, which had been used in early protocols (including UKALL I and II) lost favour since its use was associated with a decrease in dosage of other established drugs (e.g. 6MP and MTX). It has been restored as part of a third intensification module in UKALL XI (1992). Since UKALL X (1985–90) anthracycline drugs have been used at various doses in induction and intensification and concerns continue about their potential cardiotoxicity. The really late effects of these developments have yet to be fully documented. A significant proportion of long-term survivors of acute lymphoblastic leukaemia (ALL) (10–15%) will have been cured after relapse and will therefore have received significantly more treatment, including, in some cases, bone marrow transplant (BMT). They are at especially high risk of the late effects of treatment.

In acute myeloid leukaemia (AML) the situation has been different. The comparative rarity of the disease and, until recently, poor survival rate, has resulted in small numbers of survivors who received chemotherapy alone, and the opportunity to recognize late effects has been limited. Since the late 1970s increasing numbers of patients have been treated with BMT. The survivors treated by BMT (either allograft or autograft), have had a different pattern of late effects dominated by the effect of their conditioning regimen, including total body irradiation (TBI). Improved outcomes from current treatment regimens will result in more survivors who have received chemotherapy alone. The late effects will therefore differ, and so will the relative importance of anthracycline cardiotoxicity.

In non-Hodgkin's lymphoma (NHL) the treatment has changed as the nature of the disease has become better understood. Localized disease was initially treated with surgery and local, relatively high-dose radiotherapy (30–35 Gy). The survivors experienced late effects related to the anatomical site and their age at the time of treatment (survival of stage IV disease in the 1960s and 1970s was less than 10%). The subsequent recognition that this was a localized disease in only a small proportion of patients in childhood and a disseminated disease in most, resulted in increasingly intensive chemotherapy regimens. The evolution of treatment in the UK can be seen in the UKCCSG trials. In 1977 the UKCCSG 7701 trial included a randomization to establish whether adjuvant radiotherapy was necessary for all of these patients. Improved diagnostic techniques, both in imaging and in immunophenotyping allowed stratification into groups of higher risk, lower risk, B cell and T cell disease (1985, UKCCSG NHL, 8501, 02, 03). Treatment regimens have become more intensive for some, less intensive (and hopefully less damaging) for others, and more like those used for ALL (1990, UKCCSG NHL 9001, 02, 03, 04). The number of really long-term survivors has been small, and as the pattern of late effects is in a continuing state of evolution the effects which will be seen in the future will not be the same as those seen in the past.

ENDOCRINE EFFECTS, GROWTH AND FERTILITY

Growth

Impairment of growth in children treated for leukaemia has long been recognized (Sunderman and Pearson, 1969). This may be the result of a number of factors, including nutritional status, emotional stress and specific effects of therapy (Clayton et al, 1988). Radiotherapy may have a direct effect on growth as a late effect due to damage to growing bone and tissue (Probert et al, 1973). It can also lead to endocrine dysfunction if the radiation field includes the head and neck or gonads (Littley et al, 1990).

Chemotherapy

The effect of chemotherapy on growth is less clear. A comparison, between studies in Australia (Kirk et al, 1987) and Manchester (Clayton et al, 1988) of children treated for ALL with protocols, which included the same dose of cranial irradiation (2400 cGy) but different chemotherapy regimens, suggests an adverse effect on growth. The Australian children received more intensive chemotherapy both in dose and duration. The degree of growth retardation at 6 years after diagnosis expressed as mean height standard deviation score was greater in the Australian series (–1.5) than the Manchester series (–0.44). Even at 10 years, the Manchester group remained significantly less short (–0.84). Clearly, growth effects will continue to be an issue even in the absence of radiotherapy.

Irradiation

Treatment protocols for leukaemia and lymphoma in children include cranial irradiation for some patients, although the dose has varied. The hypothalamic–pituitary axis is sensitive to the effects of radiation, and the extent and nature of dysfunction is dose-dependent.

Both the hypothalamus and the pituitary can be affected by radiotherapy but the hypothalamus appears more radiosensitive and may be more affected at lower doses of radiation (2400 cGy or less). The effect of lower doses of radiation on the hypothalamus may be a subtle disturbance of the periodicity of growth hormone secretion pulses and a quantitative reduction in growth hormone secretion which may be restricted to puberty (Crowne et al, 1992; Moell et al, 1988). Survivors of standard therapy for ALL will have received a radiation dose of either 2400 cGy or 1800 cGy. At these doses the interpretation of provocation tests of GH secretion may be difficult. It has been shown that despite a normal response to provocation tests growth hormone secretion over 24 hours may be low (Blatt et al, 1984; Romshe et al, 1984).

The speed of onset of pituitary hormone deficiency is also dose-dependent. The first to appear is growth hormone (GH) deficiency (Shalet, 1982). Studies in adults (total cranial doses 3750–4250 cGy) show that the gonadotrophins and adrenocorticotrophin are the next to be affected, with secretion of thyroid-stimulating hormone (TSH) the slowest to show an effect. These studies suggest that the other hormone deficiencies may occur after a long latent period extending many years after therapy (Shalet et al, 1988).

Patients treated for relapsed ALL may have received more than one course of CNS-directed radiotherapy with cranial followed by craniospinal or TBI and will have received a much higher cumulative dose. The total cranial dose can be as high as 4800 cGy. These patients are at a considerably higher risk of long-term endocrine dysfunction and will require close monitoring.

Table 1. Dose of radiation to the hypothalamic–pituitary axis.

< 2400 cGy	At risk of early puberty, attenuated pubertal growth spurt
> 2400 cGy	At risk of early puberty, growth hormone deficiency, multiple pituitary hormone deficiency

Puberty

The timing of puberty may be affected by radiotherapy, and these children are at risk of an early or precocious puberty. There is a positive correlation between the age at pubertal onset and the age at irradiation. The youngest patients are those who are most likely to have a significant disturbance of pubertal timing following irradiation (Winter and Green, 1985; Leiper et al, 1988).

Clinical implications of cranial irradiation

The combination of growth hormone deficiency or an attenuated pubertal growth spurt together with an early onset of puberty is of considerable clinical importance. If unrecognized, it can result in loss of final height and it shortens the available time for treatment with GH. It is thus essential that this combination of problems is recognized early.

The following example illustrates the potential pitfall (Figure 1). This growth chart illustrates the effect in a female patient of the onset and treatment of ALL with an initial loss of growth velocity. The subsequent acceleration of growth is due not to catch-up growth but to the early onset of puberty and a suboptimal pubertal growth spurt. The onset of menstruation (M) heralds the closure of the epiphyses and the door is closed on treatment. The effect on final height in this situation can be severe.

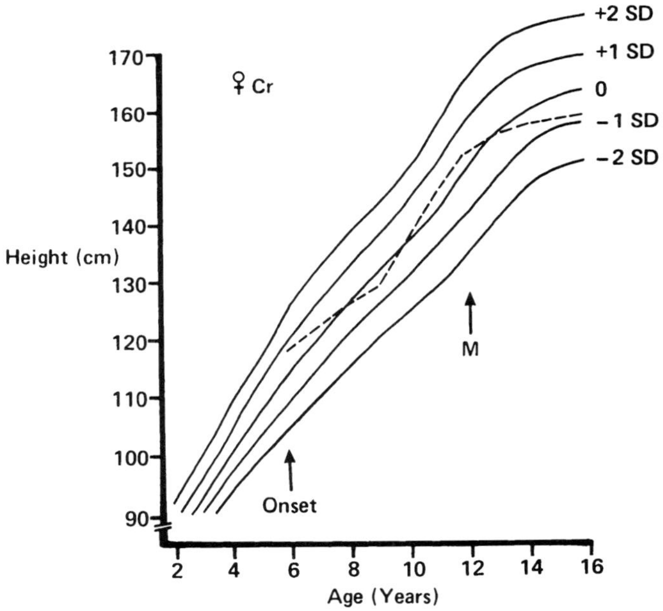

Figure 1. Growth chart of a girl who survived leukaemia, illustrating growth impairment during treatment and a subsequent suboptimal pubertal growth spurt. M indicates menarche (see text).

Deviation from an appropriate rate of growth, for an appropriate pubertal stage, at an appropriate age should alert the observer to a potential problem. This loss of harmony between the variables is a critical factor in recognizing the patient at risk. Recognition allows appropriate endocrine assessment to be performed and consideration of the use of GH. It may also be combined with a luteinizing hormone-releasing hormone (LHRH) analogue to arrest puberty and allow lengthening of the time available for GH therapy. GH, while essential for normal growth, has effects on other physiological processes. It is possible that indications for GH therapy will widen in the future and may be applicable to adult survivors of childhood malignancies.

Craniospinal irradiation

The spinal component of craniospinal irradiation results in a direct effect on the growth of the spine resulting in loss of final height. The loss of height is partly dependent on the age of the child at the time of treatment. It has been predicted that a child treated at the age of 5 might be expected to lose 7 cm from their final height and at 10 years of age 5.5 cm (Shalet et al, 1987). Although the loss is less for the older child much of the impairment occurs during puberty when maximal spinal growth occurs.

Bone marrow transplantation (BMT)

BMT is associated with abnormalities of growth (Sanders et al, 1986) primarily related to preparative regimens involving TBI (Ogilvy-Stuart et al, 1992). This may be due to a direct effect of skeletal dysplasia, GH disturbance, thyroid dysfunction, gonadal dysfunction or chronic graft-versus-host disease or its treatment. GH deficiency may occur even if the child has not previously had cranial irradiation (Borgstrom and Bolme, 1988). Effects on growth velocity are seen with both single-dose and fractionated TBI. The presence of chronic graft-versus-host disease (GVHD) worsens the problem, and, following cessation of treatment, catch-up growth is not observed despite resolution of the chronic GVHD (Sanders and Sullivan, 1989). The results of treatment with GH in this group appear to be less good but may still be helpful in reducing the severity of growth impairment. The relative insensitivity to GH may be due to the associated skeletal dysplasia (Bozzola et al, 1993). An interesting further effect of radiation on bone can be seen in the development of exostosis in the radiation field in some patients (D'Angio, 1992). These are most commonly benign osteochondromata, and in recipients of TBI they can be seen at multiple sites.

The onset of puberty is reported to be delayed or absent in some recipients of TBI but 40–50% do progress normally through puberty and do not require hormone supplementation. The presence of chronic GVHD worsens the situation and increases the proportion of recipients who demonstrate this effect (Sanders and Sullivan, 1989).

Alternative preparative regimes avoiding TBI for patients with ALL and NHL will require detailed evaluation in the future (Sanders et al, 1988).

Recommendations for follow-up

All patients require:

1. Growth charting
2. Pubertal staging, including testicular volume in boys at least 6 monthly until established normal pubertal growth spurt

More detailed endocrine assessment is required for those who are falling away from centile lines; who have suspicion of puberty prior to 9 years of age; who show loss of harmony between growth and puberty; who are already less than 10% for height; and those who have received more than 3000 cGy irradiation to the head.

Thyroid

The thyroid is extremely sensitive to the effects of irradiation and therefore even low scatter doses from adjacent fields such as spinal irradiation may lead to a significant risk of dysfunction.

Abnormalities may be seen in both secretory function and architecture with development of either benign or malignant tumours (Shalet et al, 1977; Schimpff et al, 1980). The latency period before the development of these effects may be very long. Patients who have received radiotherapy to any field with involvement of, or scatter to, the thyroid require regular monitoring of thyroid function for life and regular palpation of the gland (Shalet, 1989a). This will include those survivors of ALL and NHL who have received mediastinal, craniospinal or total body irradiation.

Biochemical monitoring is essential because of the difficulty in recognizing thyroid dysfunction clinically and the implications of an isolated raised TSH. Those with low thyroxine and raised TSH clearly need replacement therapy, but those with isolated raised TSH and normal thyroxine should receive replacement therapy sufficient to suppress the raised level (Wallace and Shalet, 1992). There is concern that an increased TSH level increases the already elevated risk of thyroid tumours in the irradiated gland (Murphy et al, 1986). In the case of an already short child, normal thyroid function should be established before any other hormone therapy is commenced.

Recommendations for follow-up

1. T4, TSH, estimation
2. Palpation of thyroid annually
   - If palpation abnormal—ultrasound scan and endocrine referral
   - TSH raised T4 normal on at least two occasions—treat with thyroxine using minimum dose necessary to restore TSH to normal. Consider trial off thyroxine after puberty is complete or after 5 years.
   - TSH raised and T4 low—treat with thyroxine, endocrine referral

Gonadal function

Gonadal function can be affected by both chemotherapy and radiotherapy in both males and females. There are, however, important differences in the sensitivity to these effects between the sexes and between different chemotherapeutic agents.

Drugs of particular concern are the alkylating agents, nitrosoureas, cytarabine and possibly cisplatinum. The effect of cyclophosphamide and cytarabine are of most concern for survivors of leukaemia and lymphoma in childhood. These effects are dose-dependent, but there is considerable individual variability in sensitivity as well as male/female variability.

Males

The function of the testis can be divided into its production of sperm (spermatogenesis) and production of steroid hormones (steroidogenesis). The Sertoli cells and germinal epithelium are responsible for spermatogenesis under the influence of follicle stimulating hormone (FSH) from the pituitary. A protein, inhibin, is also secreted by the Sertoli cells and exerts a negative feedback on the pituitary. The Leydig cells are responsible for the secretion of testosterone under the influence of luteinizing hormone (LH). Testosterone exerts its own feedback on the hypothalamus and pituitary.

Chemotherapy

Patients who have received cyclophosphamide and cytarabine may demonstrate abnormalities of spermatogenesis (Lendon et al, 1978) but not steroidogenesis (Quigley et al, 1989). The secretion of testosterone is not affected, and these patients experience normal puberty, sexual maturation and libido. They have normal LH levels but the FSH may be raised. If treatment for leukaemia and lymphoma occurs prepubertally, males who have significant gonadotoxicity will tend to have smaller testicles (12 ml or less using the Prader orchidometer). The effects of these agents on the testes may be reversible in some patients, with a recovery to fertility after a long period (Wallace et al, 1991). Patients need to be aware of this possibility! Males with raised FSH following such treatment are at risk of developing gynaecomastia, which may be embarrassing and cosmetically unacceptable.

Radiotherapy

The testis is sensitive to radiotherapy, with the effect on spermatogenesis occurring at lower exposure than the effect on secretion of testosterone (Rowley et al, 1974). The younger the child at the time of exposure the greater the risk. Patients who receive a direct dose to the testes of 2000 to 2400 cGy for testicular relapse will be rendered sterile and most will require androgen replacement therapy to allow normal pubertal development (Shalet et al, 1985).

The administration of TBI prior to bone marrow transplant, despite the lower dose to the testes, results in a high incidence of gonadal dysfunction with ablation of the germinal epithelium and almost universal sterility. Recovery has been reported in one patient 6 years after TBI (Sanders and Sullivan, 1989). Many of these patients will require androgen therapy to allow normal pubertal development. Once final height has been reached and puberty completed it may be appropriate to re-assess the need for androgen therapy as it is important to consider the need for normal libido and sexual function. Males with severe gonadal dysfunction may find their small testes cosmetically embarrassing and this may prevent involvement in activities such as swimming and may be an inhibition to normal sexual function. Testicular prosthetic implants can be offered to such patients.

Recommendations for follow-up

All patients require:

1. Growth charting
2. Pubertal staging including testicular volume in boys at least 6 monthly until established normal pubertal growth spurt
3. Semen analysis when appropriate
4. Contraception advice

Endocrine assessment is required if there are no signs of puberty by the age of 12 years, there is a reduced testicular volume in relation to pubertal stage, or there is pubertal arrest.

Females

The ovary is less sensitive to the late effects of treatment, and its ovulatory and secretory functions are closely associated. The presence of regular menses is likely to be associated with ovulatory cycles and normal sex hormone levels. Although the recipients of cyclophosphamide may have raised FSH, and oligomenorrhoea has been reported (Pasqualini et al, 1987), their prospects for fertility are better than for men (Shalet, 1989b). Those who have received radiotherapy to a region with possible scatter to the ovary, for example craniospinal, are at increased risk of significant dysfunction (Livesey and Brook, 1988).

In the largest series reported of 144 females who received TBI prior to BMT, all experienced primary ovarian failure and most developed symptoms of early menopause, but a small proportion experienced recovery of ovarian function some years later, although this was only transient in some (Sanders and Sullivan, 1989).

The effects of radiotherapy on the ovary are the result of reduction of the fixed pool of oocytes present, the number being age-dependent. The younger patient who receives a modest dose of scatter radiation to the ovaries may not manifest an early effect but may have premature ovarian failure after a period of normal ovulatory cycles (Wallace et al, 1989). A cause for concern is the possibility that female recipients of less gonadotoxic regimes may nonetheless have suffered a significant reduction in their pool of oocytes and may be at risk of premature menopause. Until more survivors reach their fourth and fifth decades this will not be clarified.

The prospects of fertility for female patients who have not received radiotherapy and are experiencing regular menses are therefore good, and there are now a considerable number of offspring to such survivors (Green et al, 1989). There is no evidence of an increased risk of germ cell mutation or other abnormalities in these offspring and as yet there is no evidence of an increased risk of cancer (Hawkins et al, 1989).

Female survivors who have received radiotherapy to fields involving the abdomen or pelvis (this includes those having craniospinal irradiation) have an increased risk of adverse outcome in pregnancy manifest as spontaneous abortion or premature labour (Li et al, 1987). It is suggested that this is due to adverse effects on the endometrium itself, uterine elasticity and uterine blood flow (Smith and Hawkins, 1989).

BMT recipients who have had TBI clearly have a risk of both uterine and ovarian failure, but a window of opportunity to become pregnant may occur for a few (Liesner et al, 1994). In the series of 144 female survivors of such a regime, three patients became pregnant on four occasions but no live births ensued (Sanders and Sullivan, 1989).

Recommendations for follow-up
All patients require:
1. Growth charting
2. Pubertal staging—at least 6 monthly until established normal pubertal growth spurt
3. Discuss
   - fertility prospects
   - contraception
   - early menopause risk
   - pregnancy prognosis

If there are no signs of puberty by the age of 11 years and the patient is considered to be at risk of ovarian dysfunction or pubertal arrest then refer for endocrine assessment.

Cardiac

Cardiac dysfunction in survivors of childhood leukaemia is uncommon. There are some groups of patients at particular risk. It is now well accepted that the cytotoxic agents known as anthracyclines can cause cardiac damage in the long term. The risk of toxicity is dose-related and exacerbated by irradiation to the heart (Steinherz et al, 1991), although it has been reported that children receiving doses as low as 45 mg/m^2 have minor abnormalities of cardiac function (Lipshultz et al, 1991). For the purposes of this review, three groups of survivors of leukaemia and lymphoma should be highlighted. (i) Survivors of acute non-lymphoblastic leukaemia who receive moderate doses of anthracyclines and who may go on to receive a bone marrow transplant (autologous or allogeneic) in which total body irradiation is used as part of the preparative regimen (Pihkala et al, 1994). (ii) Survivors of acute lymphoblastic leukaemia who are in a second or a subsequent remission. These individuals are likely to have received high doses of anthracyclines (> 300 mg/m^2; some will have had a bone marrow transplant. (iii) Patients who have had a malignant lymphoma (stage III or IV) and received anthracyclines will also be at risk of long-term problems. There is one report of cardiac dysfunction (impairment of maximal cardiac index on exercise, higher estimated posterior wall stress and pathological Q waves) following craniospinal irradiation (Jakacki et al, 1993).

Recommendations for follow-up (for full details see Steinherz et al, 1992)
All patients require:
1. Cardiac history, e.g. palpitations or chest pain
2. Annual blood pressure measurement

Patients who have received anthracyclines require:
1. Echocardiogram 1–3 months after *last* dose of anthracycline (to measure fractional shortening and left ventricular ejection fraction)
2. If normal, echocardiogram 5-yearly after last dose of anthracycline

If the dose of anthracycline exceeds 300mg/m^2, more frequent monitoring may be required. For patients who have not had an echocardiogram within 6 months of the last dose of anthracyclines, monitor 3-yearly until the growth spurt is finished. Patients receiving radiotherapy to the mediastinum have an increased risk of ischaemic heart disease; review clinically.

Genitourinary

Acute renal failure may occur at the time of presentation of leukaemia or after the onset of treatment (due to tumour lysis syndrome) but long-term renal and urinary tract abnormalities are rare. Until recently standard therapy for leukaemia and lymphoma has not included high doses of cytotoxic agents that are nephrotoxic. Systemic, moderate-dose methotrexate (6–8 g/m^2) is now used in the treatment of acute lymphoblastic leukaemia and lymphoma in the UK and USA. This drug has been reported to cause a rise in serum creatinine, but the risk is small (Seidel et al, 1994).

Renal damage can occur following a bone marrow transplant and may result from a combination of factors: total body irradiation, cyclophosphamide, long-term use of cyclosporin, nephrotoxic antibiotics and antifungal agents (e.g. amphotericin). Radiation nephritis is not thought to be a significant factor because of the relatively low dose used. Haemorrhagic cystitis is the most common toxicity seen after bone marrow transplantation in children and it may be severe.

Respiratory

Several factors relating to the treatment of leukaemia may affect lung function in the long term: a prolonged period of immunosuppression, the cytotoxic agents themselves, or radiation which may include the lungs. The use of prolonged 'maintenance' chemotherapy renders the child immunosuppressed for at least 2 years. This, in turn, leads to an increased incidence of lower respiratory tract infection (Siegel et al, 1980). In particular, opportunistic infections such as *Pneumocystis carinii* or other fungal or viral pneumonitides, may occur although the causative organism frequently goes undetected (Darbyshire et al, 1985). There are several agents that may also be implicated as a cause of pulmonary toxicity. Methotrexate is known to cause pulmonary damage in some patients; the pattern of damage appears to be idiosyncratic and is possibly immune-mediated (Sostman et al, 1976). Cyclophosphamide can cause lung fibrosis (Alvarado et al, 1978) but this is unlikely to occur following the doses used in the majority of patients with leukaemia and lymphoma. A study of a group of 69 survivors of leukaemia has demonstrated a small but significant impairment of lung function when compared with their peers. Previous chest infections, anthracyclines, bone marrow transplantation and craniospinal irradiation were all independently related to a reduction in transfer factor in survivors of leukaemia. Perhaps more interestingly, the cohort of survivors participated in significantly less regular activity than their peers, performed less well under controlled exercise conditions, and 36% of the survivors perceived themselves to be less fit than their peers (Jenney et al, 1995a).

Skin

Many patients treated with chemotherapy develop multiple pigmented naevi (Hughes and Bailey, 1989; Baird et al, 1992). This effect does not appear to be restricted to any particular drug or combination. The appearance of these naevi may be quite atypical, which leads to concern about malignancy or malignant potential. Malignant melanoma has been described as a second malignancy in association with retinoblastoma (Meadows et al, 1985) and following BMT (Sanders and Sullivan, 1989). There is clearly a possibility of interaction between genetic factors, radiotherapy and prior chemotherapy. The presence of large numbers of naevi is one of the known risk factors for malignant melanoma in the general population. Patients need to be given advice on other risk factors such as exposure to sunlight, sunburn and skin type. The aetiology is not known but may relate to immunosuppression as increased naevi have also been seen following renal transplantation and immunosuppression with cyclosporin (McGregor et al, 1991).

Radiotherapy may affect the skin, and poor or absent hair growth may occur. This is a common and distressing problem for those treated with higher doses of cranial irradiation in the past or following CNS relapse. Basal-cell naevi may occur and basal-cell carcinoma may develop in the radiotherapy field at a much younger age than in the general population.

Recommendations for follow-up

1. Inspect skin
   - especially pigmented lesions particular attention to radiotherapy fields
   - consider GVHD following allogenic BMT
2. Encourage awareness of warning changes in pigmented lesions—size, thickness, pigmentation, itching, bleeding
3. Encourage avoidance of UV exposure

Neuropsychological impairment

The introduction of CNS-directed therapy as part of the treatment for childhood leukaemia in the early 1960s dramatically improved the survival rates of children with acute lymphoblastic leukaemia. Just over 15 years later the first reports of impairment of intellectual function (e.g. memory impairment, fall in intelligence quotient (IQ)) occurring in survivors of leukaemia were published (Eiser, 1978; Meadows et al, 1981). Cranial irradiation (CRT), intrathecal methotrexate (IT-MTX) and systemic high-dose methotrexate (SYS-MTX) are used to treat occult CNS leukaemia, and some controversy exists over the extent to which each treatment modality (or even the disease itself) contributes to long-term dysfunction.

Radiation damage to the normal tissues of the central nervous system may manifest as cortical atrophy, vascular damage (mineralizing microangiopathy) or white matter destruction (leukoencephalopathy) (Price and Birdwell, 1978). A correlation between the presence of such abnormalities with long-term neuropsychological dysfunction has been reported (Brouwers et al, 1985), and there is recent evidence that calcification of the basal ganglia and/or grey or white matter junctions predicts poor intellectual and memory functioning in children surviving leukaemia during infancy (Mulhern et al, 1992).

The dose of CRT has been thought to be important in determining the severity of the impairment. One study of 35 survivors of leukaemia found that children who had received 2400 cGy had a fall in verbal IQ, and tests of reading, writing and arithmetic 10 points greater than those who had received 1800 cGy (Moore et al, 1991). Doses of 2400 cGy were used in early leukaemia trials and continue to be used if CNS disease occurs at presentation, or (in the latest MRC UK ALL trial), if the child has a high white count at diagnosis. However significant impairment of full scale intelligence quotients has also been demonstrated in a group of 203 survivors following lower doses (1800 cGy) of cranial irradiation (Jankovic et al, 1994).

An inverse relationship between the age at which the radiotherapy is administered and cognitive function has been identified (Jannoun and Chessells, 1987). It has been estimated that the mean loss of intelligence quotient scores for children treated before 4 years of age is 17 points compared with 7 for those treated after this age (Cousens et al, 1988). This, too, is controversial, and other studies have failed to find any effect of age at treatment on long-term cognitive dysfunction (Rubenstein et al, 1990).

A relationship between the time since irradiation and the degree of neuropsychological impairment has been identified, but remains controversial. In the recent study of 129 children with 1800 cGy cranial irradiation by Jankovic et al (1994), a significant decline in full-scale IQ was identified, and this increased with length of time from diagnosis. A prospective study of 24 children treated for ALL with 1800 cGy cranial irradiation also showed a decline in intellectual function with time (Rubenstein et al, 1990). Because of the concerns of late toxicity of cranial irradiation, systemic high-dose methotrexate and intrathecal MTX have been substituted in the majority of international paediatric leukaemia trials as CNS-directed therapy for those who do not have CNS disease at presentation, and are not deemed to be at 'high risk'. However, the long-term effects of these agents are not yet clear. A prospective study comparing children who have received 1800 cGy CRT and IT-MTX or SYS-MTX alone has demonstrated no significant difference between the two groups (Ochs et al, 1991). Both groups developed significant decreases in overall and verbal intelligence quotients and arithmetic achievements at a median of 6 years after cessation of treatment. Longer, prospective follow-up of all groups of children treated for leukaemia or lymphoma with CNS-directed therapy is necessary to clarify the true impact of such treatment on neuropsychological function.

Recommendations for follow-up

1. Question school/work achievements at every visit
2. Refer for psychological assessment if there is a possible problem
3. Consider associated neurological problems

Psychosocial functioning of survivors of leukaemia and lymphoma

What are the effects of a fall in IQ score or the significant disruption to family, social and school life which may occur during treatment on the long-term psychological and social functioning of the survivor? In a case–control study of educational, occupational and insurance status of 219 childhood cancer survivors (all diagnoses) in the United States, there were few differences defined between the survivors who had been treated between 1945 and 1975 and their peers, apart from a history of employment discrimination for entry into the uniformed services (Hays et al, 1992). In a similar study of patients treated more recently (1960 to 1984) there were difficulties in obtaining life insurance in 24% of those who obtained it, and the number of survivors with insurance was lower than those in the general population. The percentage of both males and females married was significantly lower than the US norms. However, the study concluded that most former paediatric cancer patients achieve adult life goals (Green et al, 1991).

However, psychological and social problems do occur, and more detailed studies of psychological functioning have also been undertaken. Perceived stress, psychological distress and lower self esteem have been demonstrated in survivors of childhood cancer (of whom almost 50% were survivors of leukaemia) (Varni et al, 1994). A study of psychological functioning of 8- to 16-year-old cancer survivors (35% had leukaemia) showed that the majority of former patients functioned within normal limits; however, as a group, they differed significantly from their peers. Those children with severe medical late effects had a poorer self concept, more depressive symptoms and a more external locus of control than those with mild to moderate late effects (Greenberg et al, 1989).

These studies demonstrate the need to monitor future cohorts of survivors continually, because as treatment protocols are modified, the long-term sequelae may change. Children at risk should be readily identified so that early steps can be taken to prevent or minimize long-term psychological problems.

Liver

Although the acute gastrointestinal toxicity of leukaemia during childhood can be severe, long-term abnormalities are rare. Liver toxicity can occur, and transient abnormalities of liver function tests have been reported following the use of methotrexate and mercaptopurine. Hepatitis B infection has been reported in older series of children with leukaemia (Vergani et al, 1982), but is now only rarely seen. The majority of children will have received several transfusions of blood products and there will be a small risk of hepatitis C or infection with the human immunodeficiency virus in patients treated before screening of blood products was introduced.

Second malignancies

A second malignancy may occur because of a genetic predisposition to cancer, the use of radiation therapy or chemotherapy (e.g. alkylating agents (Tucker et al, 1987; de Vathaire et al, 1989) or epipodophyllotoxins (Hawkins et al, 1987; Pui et al, 1991), or as a chance occurrence. The risks of developing a second primary malignancy have been determined in several cohorts of survivors but these data will continue to change (and increase) both as the therapy used in the treatment of childhood cancer changes and the length of follow-up increases. In a population-based cohort study of survivors of childhood cancer in the UK, three cases of a second malignancy were identified in survivors of leukaemia (all in the central nervous system) giving a 20-fold increase in the expected number of CNS tumours (Hawkins et al, 1987). Similar results have also been reported from the United States (Li, 1977). In a further study of 9720 children who had survived leukaemia, 43 developed a second cancer (Neglia et al, 1991). There was a seven-fold increase in all cancers, and a 22-fold increase in CNS tumours. There have been occasional reports of second cancers occurring in children who have been treated for NHL (Hawkins et al, 1987; Li, 1977); however, the overall risk of a second cancer in these children has not been defined because of the small numbers of patients at the present time.

Quality of life

The impact of the diagnosis of leukaemia and lymphoma on the quality of life of a child, adolescent or young adult is unknown. We have reviewed several areas of health in which there may be long-term abnormalities. What is not known is how much the individual survivor is affected by such sequelae of treatment. What does a loss of 7 cm in height mean to a child? What is the impact of infertility? Does the individual have long-term anxiety or depression as a result of his or her previous therapy? Several measures of health status or health-related quality of life in children are under development (Feeny et al, 1992; Jenney et al, 1995b; Eiser et al, 1995) and such measures must be validated in these patient groups. When assessing the outcome of a clinical trial, survival is clearly of utmost importance; the late effects of therapy must also be assessed, but there is also a need to ascertain the impact of therapy on the life of the child as perceived by the child.

Future implications

It is now accepted that by the end of this decade over 1 in 1000 young adults between the ages of 20 and 29 will have survived a malignancy during childhood (Meadows and Hobbie, 1986). Over 50% of these 'survivors' will have had leukaemia or a lymphoma. These facts have several implications. Although survival is paramount, it is not sufficient, and there is an urgent need to address the issues of the health and quality of life of this group of young people. Providing adequate health care for these individuals is also a challenge. As the number of survivors and age of the cohort increases, questions are raised as to who should care for them and address the unique set of problems they face. This has not yet been resolved. Many children are presently followed into adulthood by the paediatric oncologist, possibly with the support of an endocrinologist. The ideal program of long-term care has not yet been defined but it is essential that, as the numbers of survivors continue to rise, a structured programme of follow-up is provided.

Studies are under way to try to define the true incidence of long-term adverse sequelae, but prospective evaluation of the late effects of the treatment for childhood leukaemia and lymphoma is essential in future trials of therapy in order to evaluate the real costs of cure.

SUMMARY

As the survival rates of childhood leukaemia and lymphoma improve so physical, psychological and social long term effects of therapy become more apparent and more important. The late effects of therapy largely depend on the treatment the individuals have received. There are several endocrine effects of therapy, particularly growth impairment following cranial irradiation, and infertility following bone marrow transplantation. Thyroid dysfunction may also occur in patients who have received craniospinal irradiation. For patients who have received anthracyclines and/or radiotherapy to the mediastinum, long term adverse cardiac sequelae have been recognized. Other long term problems include respiratory dysfunction, genitourinary problems and perhaps most importantly adverse neuro-psychological sequelae of therapy.

Evaluation of late effects is essential so that appropriate intervention can be undertaken at an early stage with the aim of improving the quality of life of the individual in the long term. As late effects are increasingly recognized they can be anticipated and minimized. The modified need for treatment protocols to reduce late adverse sequelae (e.g. the modification of CNS directed therapy in UKALL XI) has now be recognized. However, the overall aim of therapy, that of cure, must not be compromised.

REFERENCES

Alvarado CS, Boat TF & Newman AJ (1978) Late onset pulmonary fibrosis and chest deformity in two children treated with cyclophosphamide. *Journal of Pediatrics* **92:** 443–446.

Baird EA, McHenry PM & Mackie RM (1992) Effect of maintenance chemotherapy in childhood on numbers of melanocytic naevi. *British Medical Journal* **305:** 799–801.

Blatt J, Bereu BB, Gillin JC et al (1984) Reduced pulsatile growth hormone secretion in children after therapy for acute lymphoblastic leukaemia. *Journal of Pediatrics* **104:** 182–186.

Borgstrom B & Bolme P (1988) Growth and growth hormone in children after bone marrow transplantation. *Hormone Research* **30:** 98–100.

Bozzola M, Giorgiani G, Loctelli F et al (1993) Growth in children after bone marrow transplantation. *Hormone Research* **39:** 122–126.

Brouwers P, Riccardi R, Fedio P & Poplack DG (1985) Long term neuropsychologic sequelae of childhood leukemia: correlation of CT brain abnormalities. *Journal of Pediatrics* **106:** 723–728.

Clayton PE, Shalet SM, Morris Jones PH & Price DA (1988) Growth in children treated for acute lymphoblastic leukaemia. *Lancet* **i:** 460–462.

Cousens P, Waters B, Said J & Stevens M (1988) Cognitive effects of cranial irradiation in leukaemia: a survey and meta-analysis. *Journal of Child Psychology and Psychiatry* **29:** 839–852.

Crowne EC, Wallace WHB, Moore C et al (1992) A novel variant of growth hormone (GH) insufficiency following low dose cranial irradiation. *Clinical Endocrinology* **36:** 59–68.

D'Angio GJ (1992) An overview and historical perspective of late effects of treatment for childhood cancer. In Green DM and D'Angio GJ (eds), *Late Effects of Treatment for Childhood Cancer*, pp 1–6. New York: Wiley-Liss.

Darbyshire P, Eden OB, Jameson B et al (1985) Pneumonitis in lymphoblastic leukaemia of childhood. *Pediatric Haematology and Oncology* **2:** 141–147.

de Vathaire F, Francois P, Hill C et al (1989) Role of radiotherapy and chemotherapy in the risk of second malignant neoplasms after cancer in childhood. *British Journal of Cancer* **59:** 792–796.

Eiser C (1978) Intellectual abilities among survivors of childhood leukaemia. *Archives of Diseases in Childhood* **53:** 391–395.

Eiser C, Havermans T, Craft A & Kernahan J (1995) The development of a measure to assess the perceived illness experience (PIE) following treatment for cancer. *Archives of Diseases in Childhood* **72:** 302–307.

Feeny D, Furlong W, Barr RD et al (1992) A comprehensive multiattribute system for classifying the health status of survivors of childhood cancer. *Journal of Clinical Oncology* **10:** 923–928.

Green DM, Hall B & Zevon A (1989) Pregnancy outcome after treatment for acute lymphoblastic leukaemia during childhood or adolescence. *Cancer* **64:** 2335–2339.

Green DM, Zevon MA & Hall B (1991) Achievement of life goals by adult survivors of modern treatment for childhood cancer. *Cancer* **67:** 206–213.

Greenberg HS, Kazak AE & Meadows AT (1989) Psychologic functioning in 8- to 16-year old cancer survivors and their parents. *Journal of Pediatrics* **114:** 488–493.

Hawkins MM, Draper GJ & Kingston JE (1987) Incidence of second primary tumours among childhood cancer survivors. *British Journal of Cancer* **56:** 339–347.

Hawkins MM, Draper GJ & Smith RA (1989) Cancer among 1348 offspring of survivors of childhood cancer. *International Journal of Cancer* **43:** 975–978.

Hays DM, Landsverk J, Sallan SE et al (1992) Educational, occupational and insurance status of childhood cancer survivors in their fourth and fifth decades of life. *Journal of Clinical Oncology* **10:** 1397–1406.

Hughes B & Bailey CC (1989) Excess benign melanocytic naevi. *British Medical Journal* **299:** 854–855.

Jakacki RI, Goldwein JW & Larsen RL (1993) Cardiac dysfunction following spinal irradiation during childhood. *Journal of Clinical Oncology* **11:** 1033–1038.

Jankovic M, Brouwers P, Valsecchi G et al (1994) Association of 1800 cGy cranial irradiation with intellectual function in children with acute lymphoblastic leukaemia. *Lancet* **344:** 224–227.

Jannoun L & Chessells JM (1987) Long term psychological effects of childhood leukaemia and its treatment. *Pediatric Hematology and Oncology* **4:** 293–308.

Jenney MEM, Faragher B, Morris-Jones PH & Woodcock A (1995a). Lung function and exercise capacity in survivors of childhood leukaemia. *Medical and Pediatric Oncology* **24:** 222–230.

Jenney MEM, Kane RL & Lurie N (1995b). Developing a measure of health outcomes in survivors of childhood cancer: a review of the issues. *Medical and Pediatric Oncology* **24:** 145–153.

Kirk JA, Paghurpathy P, Stevens MM et al (1987) Growth failure and growth hormone deficiency after treatment for acute lymphoblastic leukaemia. *Lancet* **i:** 190–193.

Leiper A, Stanhope R, Preece MA et al (1988) Precocious or early puberty and growth failure in girls treated for acute lymphoblastic leukaemia. *Hormone Research* **30:** 72–76.

Lendon M, Hann IM, Palmer MK et al (1978) Testicular histology after combination chemotherapy in childhood for acute lymphoblastic leukaemia. *Lancet* **ii:** 439–441.

Li FP (1977) Second malignant tumors after cancer in childhood. *Cancer* **40:** 1899–1902.

Li FP, Gimgrere K, Gelber RD et al (1987) Outcome of pregnancy in survivors of Wilms' tumor. *Journal of the American Medical Association* **257:** 216–219.

Liesner RJ, Leiper AD, Hann IM & Chessells JM (1994) Late effects of intensive treatment for acute myeloid leukaemia and myelodysplasia in childhood. *Journal of Clinical Oncology* **12:** 916–924.

Lipshultz SE, Colan SD, Gelber RD et al (1991) Late cardiac effects of doxorubicin therapy for acute lymphoblastic leukaemia in childhood. *New England Journal of Medicine* **324:** 808–815.

Littley MD, Shalet SM & Beardwell CG (1990) Radiation and hypothalamic-pituitary function. *Clinical Endocrinology and Metabolism* **4:** 147–175.

Livesey EA & Brook CGD (1988) Gonadal dysfunction after treatment of intracranial tumours. *Archives of Diseases of Childhood* **64:** 593–595.

McGregor JM, Barker JN & MacDonald DM (1991) The development of excess numbers of melanocytic naevi in an immunosuppressed identical twin. *Clinical and Experimental Dermatology* **16:** 131–132.

Meadows A & Hobbie W (1986) The medical consequences of cure. *Cancer* **58:** 524–528.

Meadows A, Gordon J, Massari D et al (1981) Declines in IQ scores and cognitive dysfunctions in children with acute lymphoblastic leukaemia treated with cranial irradiation. *Lancet* **ii:** 1015–1016.

Meadows AT, Baum E, Fossati-Bellani F et al (1985) Second malignant neoplasms in children: an update from the late effects group. *Journal of Clinical Oncology* **3:** 532–538.

Moell C, Garwicz S, Westgren U et al (1988) Blunted pubertal growth after leukaemia: a new pattern of growth hormone insufficiency. *Hormone Research* **30:** 68–71.

Moore IM, Kramer JH, Wara W et al (1991) Cognitive function in children with leukemia: effect of radiation dose and time since irradiation. *Cancer* **68:** 1913–1917.

Mulhern RK, Kovnar EH, Langston J et al (1992) Long term survivors of leukemia treated in infancy: factors associated with neuropsychological status. *Journal of Clinical Oncology* **10:** 1095–1102.

Murphy ED, Scanlon EF, Garces RM et al (1986) Thyroid hormone administration in irradiated patients. *Journal of Surgical Oncology* **31:** 214–217.

Neglia JP, Meadows AT, Robison L et al (1991) Second neoplasms after acute lymphoblastic leukemia in childhood. *New England Journal of Medicine* **325:** 1330–1336.

Ochs J, Mulhern R, Fairclough D et al (1991) Comparison of neuropsychologic functioning and clinical indicators of neurotoxicity in long-term survivors of childhood leukemia given cranial radiation or parenteral methotrexate: a prospective study. *Journal of Clinical Oncology* **9:** 145–151.

Ogilvy-Stuart AL, Clark DJ, Wallace WHB et al (1992) Endocrine deficit after fractionated total body irradiation. *Archives of Diseases in Childhood* **67:** 1107–1110.

Pasqualini T, Escobar ME, Domene H et al (1987) Evaluation of gonadal function following long-term treatment for acute lymphoblastic leukaemia in girls. *American Journal of Pediatric Hematology and Oncology* **9:** 15–22.

Pihkala J, Saarinen UM, Lundstrom U et al (1994) Effects of bone marrow transplantation on myocardial function in children. *Bone Marrow Transplantation* **13:** 149–155.

Price RA & Birdwell DA (1978) The central nervous system in childhood leukaemia III. Mineralizing microangiopathy and dystrophic calcification. *Cancer* **35:** 717–728.

Probert JC, Parker BR, Kaplan HK (1973) Growth retardation in children after megavoltage irradiation of the spine. *Cancer* **32:** 634–639.

Pui C-H, Ribeiro RC, Hancock ML et al (1991) Acute myeloid leukaemia in children treated with epipodophyllotoxins for acute lymphoblastic leukaemia. *New England Journal of Medicine* **325:** 1682–1687.

Quigley C, Cowell C, Jimenez M et al (1989) Normal or early development of puberty despite gonadal damage in children treated for acute lymphoblastic leukaemia. *New England Journal of Medicine* **321:** 143–151.

Romshe CA, Zipf WB, Miser A et al (1984) Evaluation of growth hormone release and human growth hormone treatment in children with cranial irradiation associated short stature. *Journal of Pediatrics* **104:** 177–181.

Rowley MK, Laech DR, Warner GA et al (1974) Effect of graded doses of ionising radiation on the human testis. *Radiation Research* **59:** 665–678.

Rubenstein CL, Varni JW, Katz ER (1990) Cognitive functioning in longterm survivors of childhood leukemia: a prospective analysis. *Developmental and Behavioral Pediatrics* **11:** 301–305.

Sanders J & Sullivan K (1989) Long term effects and quality of life in children and adults after marrow transplantation. *Bone Marrow Transplantation* **4:** 27–29.

Sanders JE, Pritchard S, Mahoney P et al (1986) Growth and development following marrow transplantation for leukaemia. *Blood* **68:** 1129–1135.

Sanders JE, Buckner CD, Sullivan KM et al (1988) Growth and development in children after bone marrow transplantation. *Hormone Research* **30:** 92–97.

Schimpff SC, Diggs CH, Wiswell JG et al (1980) Radiation-related thyroid dysfunction: implications for the treatment of Hodgkin's disease. *Annals of Internal Medicine* **92:** 91–98.

Seidel H, Moe PJ, Nygaard R et al (1994). Evaluation of serious adverse events in patients treated with protocols including methotrexate infusions. *Pediatric Hematology and Oncology* **11:** 165–172.

Shalet SM (1982) Growth and hormonal status of children treated for brain tumours. *Child's Brain* **9:** 284–293.

Shalet SM (1989a) Endocrine consequences of treatment of malignant disease. *Archives of Diseases in Childhood* **64:** 1635–1641.

Shalet SM (1989b) Disorders of gonadal function due to radiation and cytotoxic chemotherapy in children. *Advances in Internal Medicine and Pediatrics* **58:** 1–21.

Shalet SM, Rosenstock JD, Beardwell CG et al (1977) Thyroid dysfunction following external irradiation to the neck for Hodgkin's disease in childhood. *Clinical Radiology* **28:** 511–515.

Shalet SM, Horner A, Ahmed SR et al (1985) Leydig cell damage after testicular irradiation for lymphoblastic leukaemia. *Medical and Paediatric Oncology* **13:** 65–68.

Shalet SM, Gibson B, Swindell R et al (1987) Effect of spinal irradiation on growth. *Archives of Disease in Childhood* **62:** 461–464.

Shalet SM, Clayton PE, Price DA (1988) Growth and pituitary function in children treated for brain tumours or acute lymphoblastic leukaemia. *Hormone Research* **30:** 53–61.

Siegel SE, Nesbit ME, Baehner R et al (1980). Pneumonia during therapy for childhood acute lymphoblastic leukaemia. *American Journal of Diseases in Childhood* **134:** 28–34.

Smith RA & Hawkins MM (1989) Pregnancies after childhood cancer. *British Journal of Obstetrics and Gynaecology* **96:** 378–379.

Sostman HD, Matthay RA, Putman CE & Walker Smith GJ (1976) Methotrexate-induced pneumonitis. *Medicine* **55:** 371–388.

Steinherz LJ, Steinherz PG, Tan CTC et al (1991) Cardiac toxicity 4 to 20 years after completing anthracycline therapy. *Journal of the American Medical Association* **266:** 1672–1677.

Steinherz LJ, Graham T, Hurwitz R et al (1992). Guidelines for cardiac monitoring of children during and after anthracycline therapy: report of the cardiology committee of the Children's Cancer Study Group. *Pediatrics* **89:** 942–949.

Sunderman CR & Pearson HA (1969) Growth effects of long-term antileukaemia therapy. *Journal of Pediatrics* **75:** 1058–1062.

Tucker MA, Meadows AT & Boice JD (1987) Leukemia after therapy with alkylating agents for childhood cancer. *Journal of the National Cancer Institute* **78:** 459–464.

Varni JW, Katz ER, Colegrove R & Dolgin M (1994) Perceived stress and adjustment of long term survivors of childhood cancer. *Journal of Psychosocial Oncology* **12:** 1–16.

Vergani D, Locasciulli A, Masera A et al (1982) Histological evidence of hepatitis-B-virus infection with negative serology in children with acute leukaemia who develop chronic liver disease. *Lancet* **i:** 361–364.

Wallace WHB & Shalet SM (1992) Growth and endocrine function following treatment of childhood malignant disease. In Plowman PN and Pinkerton CR (eds) *Paediatric Oncology. Clinical Practice and Controversies*, pp 531–557. London: Chapman and Hall Medical.

Wallace WHB, Shalet SM, Hendry JH et al (1989) Ovarian failure following abdominal irradiation in childhood: the radiosensitivity of the human oocyte. *British Journal of Radiology* **62:** 995–998.

Wallace WHB, Shalet SM, Lendon M & Morris Jones PH (1991) Male fertility in long-term survivors of acute lymphoblastic leukaemia in childhood. *International Journal of Andrology* **14:** 312–319.

Winter RJ & Green OC (1985) Irradiation-induced growth hormone deficiency: blunted growth response and accelerated skeletal maturation to growth hormone therapy. *Journal of Pediatrics* **106:** 609–612.

6

The role of high-dose chemoradiotherapy and bone marrow transplantation in childhood leukaemia and lymphoma

KENT A. ROBERTSON
FRANKLIN O. SMITH

Bone marrow transplantation (BMT) for acute leukaemias and lymphomas has undergone significant evolution over the past two decades. As initially attempted, marrow transplantation served only as a form of salvage therapy for patients with end-stage or refractory disease (Thomas et al, 1977). Its use has since evolved to the point where it is widely considered to be the primary mode of therapy for children with acute myelogenous leukaemia (AML) in first clinical remission (CR) who have HLA-identical family donors, in children with acute lymphoblastic leukaemia (ALL) or lymphoma beyond first CR, and in children with high-risk ALL in first CR.

ACUTE MYELOID LEUKAEMIA

The treatment of the heterogeneous group of diseases classified as the acute myeloid leukaemias has undergone tremendous improvement over the past several decades. Approximately 75% of children diagnosed with AML will enter a complete clinical remission with long-term, disease-free survival in 30–40% of these children (Amadori et al, 1993; Woods et al, 1993; Wells et al, 1994).

The treatment of childhood AML has traditionally been divided into three phases: remission induction followed by consolidation therapy (chemotherapy versus autologous marrow transplantation versus allogeneic marrow transplantation) and then maintenance in those patients who do not receive BMTs. The first report of BMT in children with AML in first remission was by Sanders et al (1985). In this study, 38 children with AML in first CR received HLA-matched sibling BMTs following cyclophosphamide and total body irradiation (TBI). The probability of disease-free survival (DFS) reached a plateau of 64% at 3 years with relapse in 5 of 38 patients being the most frequent cause of death. These findings were supported by a Childrens Cancer Group study (1979–83) which demonstrated a superior outcome for patients receiving HLA-matched sibling

Baillière's Clinical Paediatrics—
Vol. 3, No. 4, November 1995
ISBN 0-7020-2075-3

transplants compared with those patients receiving chemotherapy only (survival: 50% versus 36% at 5 years) (Nesbit et al 1994).

More recently, the Childrens Cancer Group examined whether HLA-matched sibling marrow transplantation was superior to high-dose chemotherapy alone (Wells et al, 1994). Following remission induction, children underwent a 'biological' randomization to allogeneic marrow transplantation following TBI (2.0 Gy twice daily for 3 days) and cyclophosphamide (120 mg/kg) if an HLA-identical sibling donor was available. Overall, 96 children received a BMT and 343 received chemotherapy only. When the analysis of survival and DFS was based upon the biological randomization (HLA donor, $n = 113$; no donor, 298) there was no difference in survival (52 versus 46% at 5 years) or DFS (46 versus 36%) for patients with an HLA-matched donor compared to patients without a donor. When outcome was determined according to the therapy actually received (BMT, $n = 96$; chemotherapy alone, $n = 343$) or for the subgroup of patients who were correctly treated (BMT, $n = 92$; chemotherapy alone, $n = 297$), BMT was superior to chemotherapy with regard to DFS (54 versus 37% at 5 years), but there was no difference with regard to overall survival (54 versus 45% at 5 years). This large, cooperative group study illustrates the complex nature of the study designs and statistical analyses required for the interpretation of the results of different treatment modalities.

The Asociazione Italiana Ematologia ed Oncologia Pediatrica Cooperative Group reported allogeneic BMT to be superior over chemotherapy alone (Amadori et al 1993). In their study, 161 children with newly diagnosed AML received induction chemotherapy with cytarabine and daunorubicin followed by daunorubicin, cytarabine and thioguanine (DAT) consolidation therapy. Patients were assigned to receive an allogeneic BMT if an HLA-identical sibling was available, or randomized to receive three additional courses of DAT as post-remission chemotherapy or autologous BMT. The 5-year DFS of 51% for patients in the allogeneic BMT group was superior to the 21% DFS for autologous BMT patients and 27% DFS for patients who received chemotherapy alone ($P = 0.03$).

Despite these studies demonstrating the apparent superiority of BMT over chemotherapy for children with AML in first CR, some groups raise concerns of possible selection bias in favour of transplanted children (Pinkel, 1993) and the failure of randomized trials to demonstrate superiority of transplant over intensive chemotherapy when outcome is measured by intent-to-treat rather than the treatment actually delivered (Santos, 1992). Transplant-related mortality has also contributed to the debate regarding the superiority of BMT. However, with improved supportive care measures, transplant-associated mortality continues to decrease. In a French study over a period of 11 years, 74 children with AML in first CR received HLA-identical, related marrow transplants after conditioning regimens containing TBI ($n = 54$) or busulfan ($n = 20$) (Michel et al, 1992). When the results were analysed according to the three time periods in which transplantation occurred (1979–1982, 1983–1986, 1987–1990), probabilities of event-free survival (EFS) were 43, 48 and

82% respectively ($P < 0.02$) with transplant-related mortality probabilities of 36, 36 and 3% respectively ($P < 0.01$). Multivariate analysis identified the absence of acute graft-versus-host disease (GVHD) and the year of transplantation as the two factors which had a favourable impact upon outcome. Some chemotherapy-only studies have also yielded good outcomes—such as the AML-BFM-83 non-randomized study of intensive chemotherapy for treatment of children with AML in first CR, where an EFS rate of 45% at 6 years was reported (Creutzig et al, 1990). Unfortunately, the issue is further confused by the BFM's subsequent study, AML-BFM-87, which could not reproduce the earlier result, attributing the earlier success to the use of prophylactic cranial irradiation (Creutzig et al, 1993).

BMT has also been successful for patients who fail to achieve a first remission, with 30–50% of patients being alive and disease free 3 months to 11 years following transplantation (Zander et al, 1985; Clift et al, 1987; Forman et al, 1991). Few studies have been reported for children with AML in relapse or beyond first remission. Brochstein et al reported the results of 38 children with AML in relapse or first, second, or third remission who received HLA-compatible sibling BMTs following hyperfractionated TBI (11 doses of 120 cGy) and cyclophosphamide 120 mg/kg (Brochstein et al 1987) For patients receiving BMTs in first remission, the probability of DFS was approximately 65%, 75% for patients in second CR, and 33% for patients in third CR or relapse at the time of transplantation (Figure 1). Unlike patients with advanced stage disease, the probability of relapse was extremely small for patients transplanted in first CR.

In 1977, Gorin et al (1977) reported the first successful autologous marrow transplant (ABMT) for AML. Studies of ABMT for patients with AML are difficult to interpret for a variety of issues, including small sample sizes, variable durations of remission at the time of transplantation, wide age range of patients reported, the type and intensity of previous chemotherapy regimens, the use of purged and unpurged marrow, and the purging method utilized. Additionally, the use of ABMT for AML has been considered by many investigators to be problematic because of prolonged time to engraftment, the lack of a graft-versus-leukaemia effect, and concern over residual leukaemia cells in the infused marrow.

While ABMT has proven to be an effective form of therapy for some patients with AML (Woods et al, 1993; Tiedemann et al, 1993), it appears to be only minimally superior to chemotherapy alone. Autologous transplant appears to be equal to, or slightly worse than, allogeneic transplant for children with AML in first CR. In the Childrens Cancer Group pilot study 2861, children received 4-hydroperoxycyclophosphamide (4-HC) purged autologous marrow grafts ($n = 58$) or HLA-matched sibling allogeneic marrow ($n = 16$) after a preparative regimen of busulfan and cyclophosphamide (Woods et al, 1993). At 3 years, the probability of DFS was 51% for children receiving 4-HC-purged autologous grafts versus 55% for those patients receiving allogeneic transplants ($P = 0.92$) (Figure 2). In a study of similar size, Amadori et al reported 24 children who received allogeneic transplants after conditioning with cyclophosphamide and total

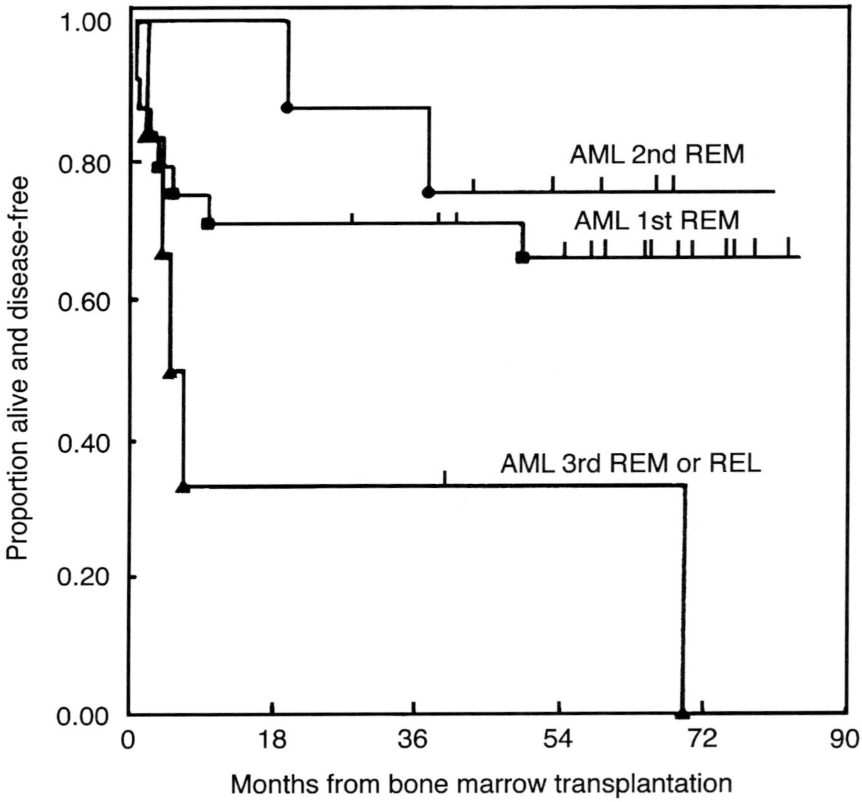

Figure 1. Disease-free survival among children receiving transplants for AML. Twenty-four patients received transplants in first remission (REM), 8 in second remission, and 6 in either third remission or relapse (REL). From Brochstein et al (1987, *New England Journal of Medicine* **317:** 1618–1624) with permission.

body irradiation and 35 children who received unmodified autologous marrow after a preparative regimen of carmustine, amsacrine, etoposide, and cytarabine (BAVC) (Amadori et al, 1993). The group of patients who received allogeneic transplants had a superior outcome with a DFS probability of 51% compared with 21% for autologous patients ($P = 0.03$). However, the apparent superiority of allogeneic transplantation in this study is complicated by the fact that two dramatically different conditioning regimens were used.

A recent report by Tiedemann et al showed a 5-year EFS rate of 68% from the time of diagnosis and 87% following ABMT for a group of 31 children with AML in first CR who had received intensive pre-transplant cytoreduction followed by a preparative regimen of high-dose melphalan (Tiedemann et al, 1993). Only 3 children had relapsed at a minimal follow-up time of 25 months. These impressive results were attributed to the use

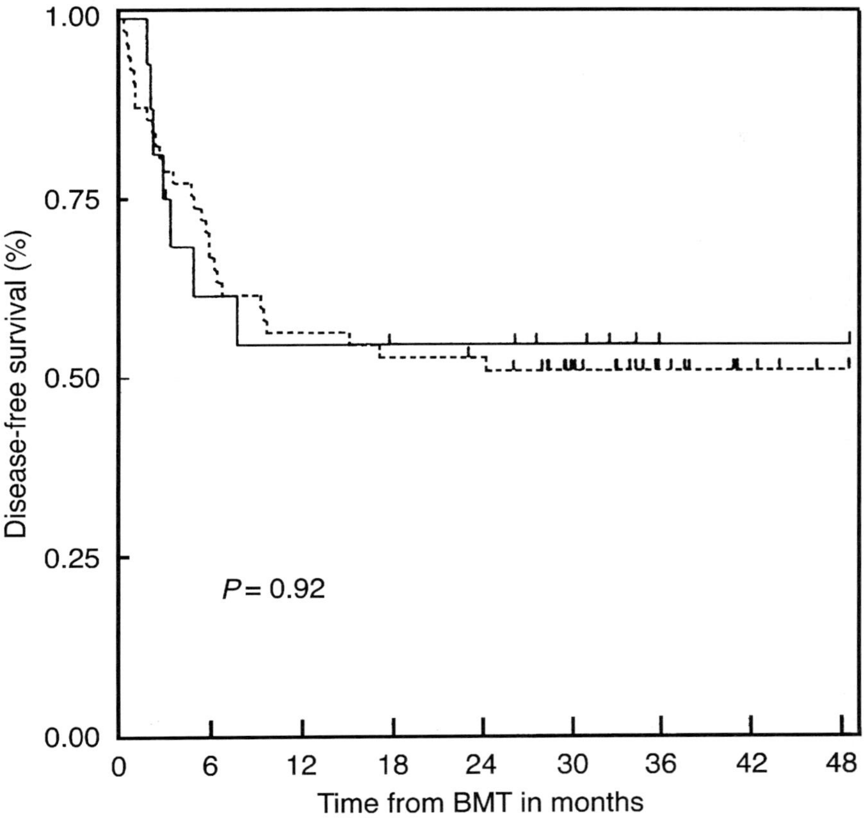

Figure 2. Log-rank DFS from the day of transplant for 58 patients undergoing autologous BMT (dashed line) and 16 patients undergoing allogeneic BMT (solid line) after achieving remission on CCG-2861. From Woods et al (1993, *Journal of Clinical Oncology* **11:** 1448–1457) with permission.

of high-dose melphalan and to the method of marrow separation and stem cell enrichment using a discontinuous percoll gradient which may have resulted in a greater depletion of contaminating AML blasts. The presence of AML blasts in autologous marrow grafts remains a major concern. It has been shown in recent gene-marking studies that autologous marrow contributed to the relapse of disease in two patients who underwent ABMT for AML in remission (Brenner at al, 1993). Several methods have been used to purge leukaemic blasts from the marrow with the cyclophosphamide analogue, 4-HC, the most widely used, although 4-HC as well as other purging modalities have not yet been demonstrated to be efficacious.

While allogeneic marrow transplants are associated with a lower rate of relapse, possibly as a result of the graft-versus-leukaemia effect, allogeneic transplantation is associated with higher mortality due in large part to graft-versus-host disease. In contrast, autologous transplants are associated with lower transplant-related mortality, but do have higher rates of relapse due to the absence of a graft-versus-leukaemia effect or the presence of contaminating leukaemia cells in the infused marrow or both. Newer strategies are needed to address these issues.

ACUTE LYMPHOCYTIC LEUKAEMIA

Childhood ALL is one of the most treatable forms of cancer, with EFS rates for newly diagnosed ALL currently in the range 60–75% (Pui and Crist, 1994). Because conventional chemotherapy strategies have been so successful in the treatment of childhood ALL, high-dose chemoradiation therapy followed by stem cell rescue has been used primarily for children with high-risk disease in first remission or for the treatment of children beyond first remission.

While most children who sustain a relapse of their leukaemia will achieve a second remission with chemotherapy, the treatment of choice for their subsequent therapy has been a subject of some controversy. The majority of studies of children treated with chemotherapy alone for ALL in second remission report EFS rates of 10–20% (Henze et al, 1991; Sadowitz et al, 1993). The duration of first remission appears to an important factor in determining the likelihood of inducing long-term, disease-free survival following initial relapse, with children who have short periods of remission (generally < 36 months) having a worse outcome. Therefore, marrow transplantation has primarily been utilized for those high-risk children who have first remissions of < 36 months or who relapse while receiving therapy.

The duration of first remission has also been an important factor in predicting outcome after allogeneic marrow transplantation (Brochstein et al, 1987; Barrett et al, 1994), with improved survival for those children whose first remissions are greater than 36 months. The role of HLA-matched sibling marrow transplantation for children with ALL in second CR was recently addressed by Barrett et al (1994). In this study, the results of marrow transplantation for 255 children who received HLA-matched sibling transplants as reported to the International Bone Marrow Transplant Registry (IBMTR) were compared in a matched-pair fashion to 255 similar children who received chemotherapy on Pediatric Oncology Group protocols. This analysis demonstrated that DFS at 5 years was higher after matched sibling transplantation than after chemotherapy (40 versus 17%, $P < 0.001$) (Figure 3) with the probability of relapse lower among patients who received transplants (45 versus 80%, $P < 0.001$). The apparent superiority of transplantation was demonstrated for patients who had first remissions of less than 36 months as well as for those patients whose initial remission was greater than 36 months. Given the limitations of this type of analysis, this study strongly suggests that bone marrow transplants from HLA-identical siblings results in improved DFS with a lower probability of relapse.

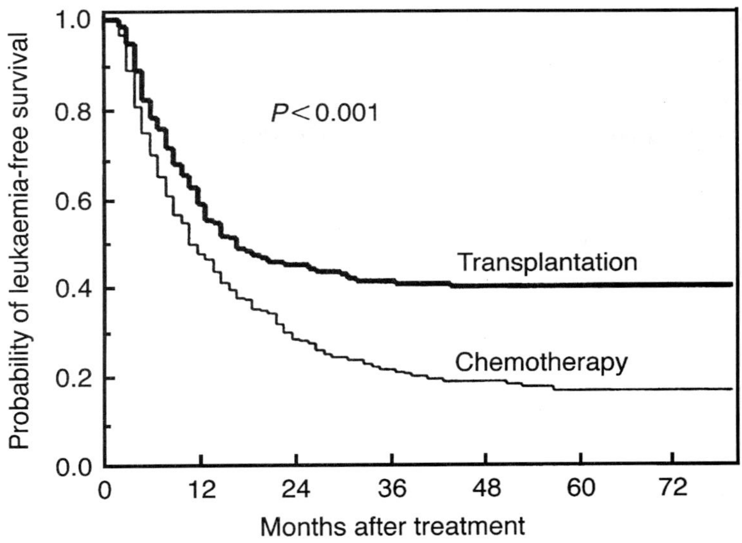

Transplantation	255	133	81	60	47	37	28
Chemotherapy	255	105	58	39	29	19	15

Figure 3. Actuarial probability of leukaemia-free survival in matched cohorts of children receiving chemotherapy or undergoing transplantation. The numbers below the figure indicate the numbers of children at risk. From Barrett et al (1994, *New England Journal of Medicine* **331:** 1253–1258) with permission.

Sanders et al (1987) have reported similar results for 57 children with ALL in second CR who received HLA-identical sibling transplants after conditioning with cyclophosphamide and TBI. In this study of children who had initial remissions of less than 36 months, the DFS was 40% with a plateau extending from 2.5 to 10.4 years. Unfortunately, some children will not enter a second remission and of those who do, only a minority of children will have a suitably matched, related marrow donor (Graham-Pole, 1989). Therefore, alternative sources of stem cells may be considered for transplantation, including purged autologous marrow, mismatched related donors, and matched unrelated marrow donors, although there are few data in the literature regarding the latter two sources in children.

While most studies utilizing autologous marrow have employed immunological or pharmacological methods of purging to eliminate residual leukaemia cells in the graft, the efficacy of purging has not been demonstrated for the acute leukaemias. The use of purged autologous marrow transplantation for children with ALL has been widely explored, with EFS rates of approximately 20% generally reported (Kersey et al, 1987). Sallan et al (1989) reported a 2-year DFS rate of 29% for 44 children with ALL beyond first CR who received purged autologous transplants with a DFS rate of only 10% in patients who relapsed after an initial remission of less than 24 months compared to a DFS probability of 51% for patients whose first remission was greater than 24 months. This work has been extended by Billet et al (1993) to now include 51 children with ALL beyond first CR whose duration of first remission was greater than 24 months. These children received CALLA (CD10)-purged autologous marrow grafts after conditioning with cytarabine, teniposide, cyclophosphamide and TBI. The DFS at 3 years was an impressive 58%, with 27 of 51 children alive in continuous CR at a median of 39 months post-transplant (Figure 4).

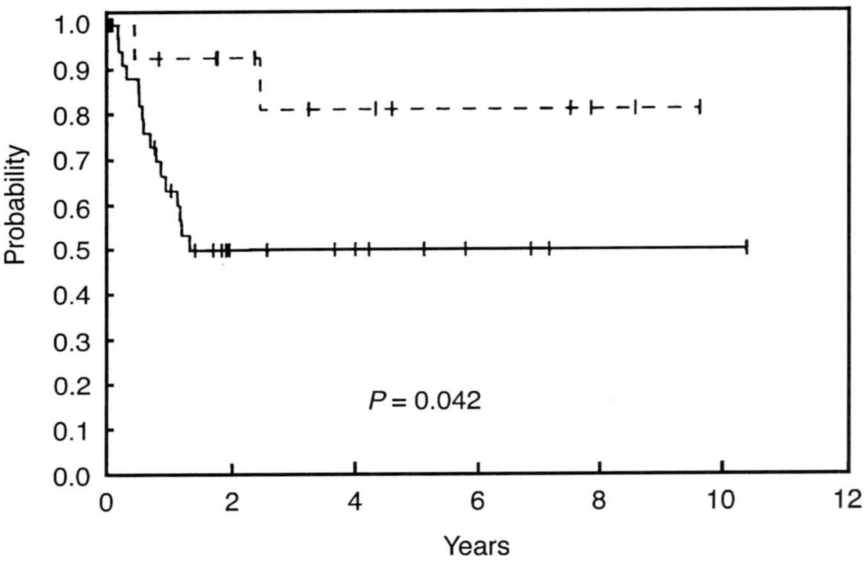

Figure 4. Kaplan-Meier plot of leukaemia-free survival by longest remission: 24 to 48 months (solid line) versus greater than 48 months (dashed line). Tick marks represent individual patients continuing at risk. From Billet et al (1993, *Blood* **81:** 1651–1657) with permission.

For children with ALL with high-risk features, transplantation in first CR may be beneficial. Approximately 5% of children with ALL have the Philadelphia chromosome (Ph+) with the t(9;22) cytogenetic abnormality. While most of these children will enter an initial remission, most will relapse resulting in a poor outcome. Barrett et al (1992) reported the results of 67 matched sibling transplants for Ph+ ALL that were reported to the IBMTR. They found a 2-year probability of DFS of 38% for patients transplanted in first CR, 41% for patients transplanted after relapse of their disease, and 25% for patients who were transplanted after failing induction chemotherapy.

CHRONIC MYELOGENOUS LEUKAEMIA

Chronic myelogenous leukaemia (CML) is a clonal panmyelopathy which accounts for approximately 3–5% of childhood leukaemia. This disease arises from neoplastic transformation of a pluripotent stem cell characterized by a reciprocal translocation of chromosomes 9q and 22q, commonly known as the Philadelphia chromosome. As in adults, the chronic phase of the disease always evolves to a more aggressive and usually drug-resistant blastic phase. Although treatment of patients in the chronic phase of CML can produce median survivals of 60–65 months (Kantarjian et al, 1993), cure of disease is achieved only by BMT.

A report of adult and paediatric patients with CML from the International Bone Marrow Transplant Registry showed that the probability of survival 3 years after matched-sibling BMT while in chronic, accelerated, or blast phase was 63, 36 and 12%, respectively (Speck et al, 1985). Similar results for adults and children have been reported utilizing matched and mismatched unrelated marrow donors (Beatty et al, 1989; McGlave et al, 1990), with McGlave et al reporting an actuarial DFS rate of 29% at 2.5 years.

Factors that have been shown to have prognostic significance include the phase of disease, time interval between diagnosis and marrow transplantation, and of particular importance to children, younger at the time transplant (< 20–30 years of age) (Thomas et al, 1986; Thomas and Clift, 1989; McGlave, et al 1987). Gamis et al (1993) reported 11 children with CML in chronic or accelerated phase who received unmodified marrow transplants from unrelated or matched sibling donors after cyclophosphamide and TBI conditioning. Late graft failure and severe acute GVHD was more problematic in unrelated donor grafts. The Kaplan-Meier estimate for DFS at 3 years was not statistically different for patients receiving matched sibling grafts versus unrelated donor grafts (78 versus 45%, $P = 0.09$) (Figure 5). Similarly, relapse rates were not significantly different between the two groups. Klingebiel et al (1990) reported 14 paediatric patients with CML in chronic or accelerated phase who received HLA-identical or 1 antigen mismatched related or unrelated marrow grafts after conditioning with cyclophosphamide and TBI with or without etoposide, or cyclophosphamide and busulfan. Only two children died of transplant-related complications, with one child having relapse of disease. The probability of DFS at 5.5 years post-transplant was 61%, suggesting that allogeneic marrow transplantation for children is relatively safe and effective therapy for CML.

Transplantation of autologous marrow for CML has been attempted to expand the use of BMT for patients who do not have allogeneic or syngeneic donors (Haines et al, 1984; Reiffers et al, 1991). Many of these patients had a cytogenetic conversion post-transplant with a second chronic phase achieved and survival that appeared to be longer than for patients who did not receive autografts. Unfortunately, these patients had recurrent blast transformation within 1 year of initial transformation. This experience suggested that autologous transplantation may be of limited value because

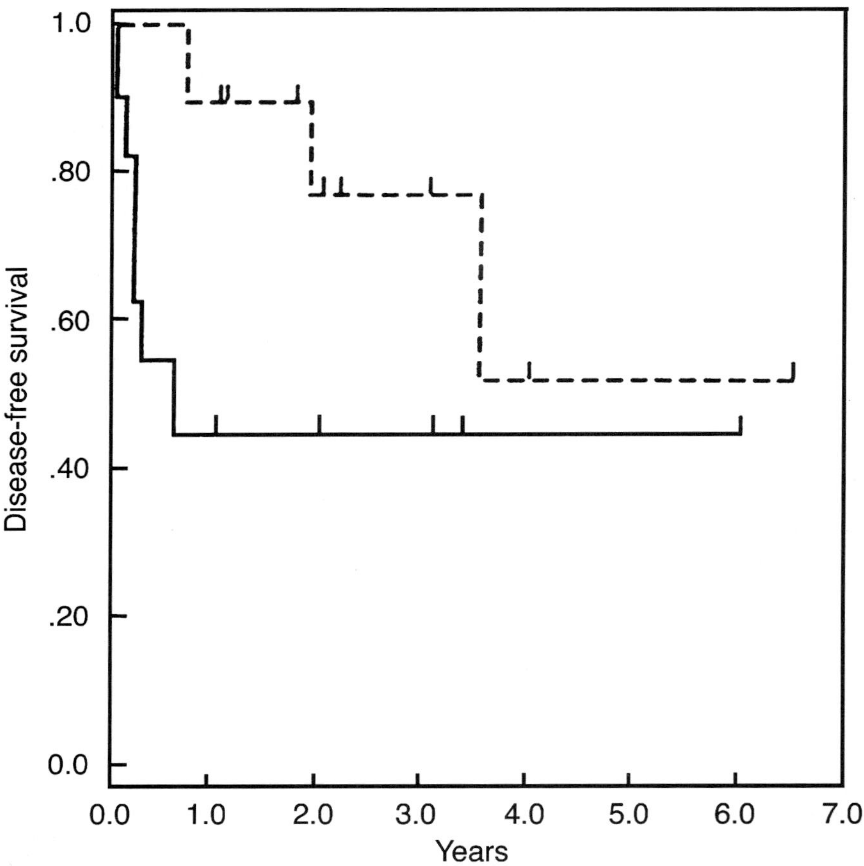

Figure 5. Kaplan-Meier estimated DFS curves for the unrelated donor ($n = 11$, solid line) and matched sibling donor ($n = 11$, dashed line) groups ($P = 0.09$). From Gamis et al (1993, *Journal of Clinical Oncology* **11:** 834–838) with permission.

of the infusion of leukaemic precursor cells in the stored autologous marrow. Infused marrow may give rise to relapse as demonstrated in recent studies of retrovirally marked CML marrow (Deisseroth et al, 1994). Coulmbel et al (1983) demonstrated that the marrow of patients with chronic phase CML contains normal haematopoietic precursor cells that display a selective growth advantage over leukaemic precursor cells in long-term culture systems. This finding has been successfully exploited to treat patients with CML with autologous marrow following in vitro long-term culture (Barnett et al, 1989).

More recently, Carella et al (1993) have reported the use of intensive chemotherapy for cytoreduction and peripheral blood stem cell mobilization for patients with chronic or accelerated phase of CML who did not have allogeneic donors. Patients whose peripheral blood stem cells were collected within 2 years of diagnosis or in chronic phase were more likely to have Philadelphia chromosome negative (Ph–) collections than those patients who were collected more than 2 years from diagnosis or who were in accelerated phase. Nine patients were transplanted with Ph(–) peripheral blood stem cells after a conditioning regimen of cyclophosphamide and TBI. Two patients failed to engraft, and one patient died of infectious complications. Five patients had sustained remissions of 3–19 months post-transplant, with two patients having recurrent leukaemia at 3 and 7 months post-transplant.

The European Group for Bone Marrow Transplantation reported 49 adult patients with CML in chronic phase who underwent autologous peripheral blood stem cell transplantation or autologous marrow transplantation (Reiffers et al, 1994). Of the 39 patients who had a complete haematological response, 34 were alive 17–52 months post-transplant. Of 34 patients, 15 had a major response, with >65% Ph(–) metaphases. The probability of transformation at 3 years was 28%, with a probability of survival of 81%. These studies suggests that autologous PBSC transplantation is a potentially curative mode of therapy for some patients with CML without an available donor.

JUVENILE CHRONIC MYELOGENOUS LEUKAEMIA

Juvenile chronic myelogenous leukaemia (JCML) is a rare myeloproliferative disease of childhood which is commonly associated with neurofibromatosis type 1 and abnormalities of chromosome 7. Affected children demonstrate fever, bleeding, frequent infections, failure to thrive, skin rashes, lymphadenopathy, and hepatosplenomegaly. Laboratory findings include anaemia, elevated white blood cell counts with immature monocytes and myeloid cells and occasional blasts, elevations of fetal haemoglobin, thrombocytopenia and elevated plasma triglycerides. While bone marrow transplantation has been demonstrated to be curative (Sanders et al, 1988; Smith et al, 1994), conventional use of chemotherapy has not proven to be beneficial, with median survivals of 1–2 years (Chan et al, 1987). However, Castleberry et al (1994) recently reported the use of isotretinoin (13-cis-retinoic acid) for the treatment of 10 newly diagnosed JCML patients. In this group of patients, two children had complete responses, three had partial responses, and one had a minimal response, while four children had progressive disease while on therapy. Three of the four complete or partial responders did not receive a bone marrow transplant and are alive 36–83 months following diagnosis.

Smith et al (1994) have recently reported the results of allogeneic marrow transplantation for a large group of children with JCML. In this series, 27 children received marrow from HLA-matched siblings, 1, 2 or 3 antigen mismatched family members, or unrelated donors following conditioning with a variety of preparative regimens. Five patients were reported to survive disease-free 2.7–10 years (median, 7.3 years), with ten patients having relapse of their disease 1.6–56 months (median, 2.8 months) following transplantation. Kaplan-Meier estimates for DFS, relapse and non-relapse mortality at 5 years post-transplant were 25, 49 and 44% respectively. Overall, these results suggest that BMT may be curative for some patients with JCML, but that relapse is still the most frequent cause of death.

HODGKIN'S DISEASE

The majority of children with Hodgkin's disease (HD) will be cured of their disease with non-transplant therapy. The Stanford group reported 57 children with HD (≤17 years of age) treated with chemoradiation therapy (Hunger et al, 1994). Children with stage I–III disease had 10-year DFS of 100%, while those with stage IV disease had DFS of 69%. Current efforts are being directed toward reducing therapy for those with good-risk disease while intensifying therapy for high-risk disease. It is those patients with high risk or relapsed disease that may benefit from marrow transplantation.

Since relatively few paediatric patients receive transplants for HD, most transplant centres include paediatric patients in with adult protocols. In a review of 1007 patients transplanted for HD, the European Bone Marrow Transplant Group Lymphoma Registry examined the outcome of 81 paediatric patients (< 16 years of age) compared to 81 case matched adults patients (> 16 years of age). No statistically significant differences were found between the paediatric and adult groups, with 36 of 81 paediatric patients and 37 of 81 adult patients surviving progression-free with a median follow-up of 34 months (Williams et al, 1993). Thus, conclusions drawn in transplant studies for HD in mixed paediatric/adult trials are generally applicable to both populations. Most series reported have about 25–35% young adults (≤ 21 years of age).

Patients with relapsed HD are at high risk of treatment failure. Risk factors that contribute to their outcome include (in order of increasing risk) a CR ≤ 12 months, refractory disease initially, and multiply relapsed disease. Conventional chemoradiotherapy will salvage some of these patients with DFS of 38–48% (Tourani et al, 1992; Fuchs et al, 1994). Initial transplant studies for patients with multiply relapsed HD showed the feasibility of ABMT to yield long-term DFS in some of these extremely high-risk patients (10–30%). More recently, salvage chemotherapy was compared to ABMT in a randomized prospective fashion by the British National Lymphoma Investigation group (Linch et al, 1993). Patients with relapsed HD were assigned to receive carmustine (BCNU), etoposide (VP-16), cytarabine (Ara-C), and melphalan (BEAM) followed by ABMT or a lower dose of the same chemotherapy not requiring ABMT (mini-BEAM). Twenty patients were treated on each arm with a 34-month progression-free survival rate of 53% for those receiving ABMT compared to 10% for those receiving mini-BEAM. This study demonstrated the usefulness of ABMT over conventional chemotherapy for allowing dose escalation with a direct therapeutic benefit.

Chemotherapy dose escalation and transplantation early after relapse are important factors for improving transplant outcome. Armitage and his colleagues in Nebraska used a transplant preparative regimen of cyclophosphamide, BCNU, and etoposide (CBV) for treating relapsed HD, and achieved an overall 4 year DFS of 27%. The DFS for patients who failed 1, 2 or 3 chemotherapy regimens before transplant was 44, 33 and 21% respectively (Armitage et al, 1991). A similar group of relapsed HD patients received ABMTs by the Vancouver transplant group with intensified dosing of CBV resulting in an overall DFS of 47% after 5 years but at the cost of 21% toxic deaths (Reece et al, 1991). Other studies have shown similar results with various preparative regimens (see Table 1).

Table 1. Bone marrow transplantation for Hodgkin's disease.

Reference	Number of patients	Treatment regimen[1]	DFS[2]/Follow-up
Armitage et al, 1991	70	CBV	27%/4 years
Reece et al, 1991	56	CBV	47%/5 years
Linch et al, 1993	20	BEAM	53%/3 years
Chopra et al, 1993	156	BEAM	50%/5 years
Crump et al, 1993	73	etopside, melphalan	38%/4 years
Yahalom et al, 1993	47	TLI, etoposide, cyclophosphamide	50%/6.5 years
Spinolo et al, 1993	21	CBV + P	29%/3 years
Reece et al, 1994	58	CBV ± P	64%/2.3 years

[1] CBV, cyclophosphamide, BCNU (carmustine), etoposide (VP-16); BEAM, BCNU, etoposide, cytosine arabinoside, melphalan; TLI, total lymphoid irradiation; P, cisplatin.
[2] DFS, disease-free survival.

Most recently, the Vancouver group (Reece et al, 1994; Bierman et al, 1994), modified their approach to ABMT for HD with improved results. First, they treated patients ($n = 58$) in first relapse who had failed only a single chemotherapeutic regimen. Second, they dose intensified the CBV + cisplatin regimen over that reported earlier (Spinolo et al, 1993), but moderated the dose of BCNU from their previous series of patients (Reece et al, 1991). Third, nearly all patients received re-induction with chemotherapy and/or radiation prior to receiving their conditioning regimen and ABMT. The overall disease free survival was 64%. In the analysis of their data, they identified three risk factors, including remission < 1 year, extra-nodal disease at relapse, and 'B' symptoms (fever, night sweats, weight loss). They found that patients with none of the risk factors had a 3-year DFS of 100%, while those with one risk factor had a DFS of 81%, and 40% DFS for those with two risk factors, and 0% for patients with all three risk factors. There were only three toxic deaths (6.6%) compared with their previous series noted above. This study demonstrates the benefit of ABMT for patients in first relapse.

There have been relatively few studies of the role of allogeneic BMT in relapsed HD, but of those reported, there appears to be evidence for a graft-versus-lymphoma effect. Studies from Johns Hopkins showed a 17–24% lower relapse rate in patients receiving allogeneic BMTs compared to

ABMT for relapsed HD, although this was offset by an increased transplant-related mortality (Jones et al, 1991). The Seattle transplant group reported 127 patients with very high risk or end-stage HD that underwent allogeneic or autologous BMT (Anderson et al, 1993). Twelve of 44 patients receiving HLA-matched sibling BMTs (26%) survive disease free compared to 14 of 68 patients receiving ABMT (14%) surviving without disease with a follow-up of 5 years. The significantly lower relapse rate ($P = 0.05$) in the patients receiving matched sibling allogeneic BMTs (45%) compared to ABMT (76%) suggests a graft-versus-lymphoma effect with no difference in transplant related mortality. An additional source of marrow stem cells for patients with marrow involvement by their disease or prior pelvic radiation without a matched sibling donor is autologous peripheral blood stem cells. There are reports of good engraftment and DFS of 34–64% after 5 years (Haas et al, 1992; Kessinger et al, 1992).

NON-HODGKIN'S LYMPHOMA

The results of conventional therapy with non-Hodgkin's lymphoma (NHL) are excellent. A recent report from the Berlin–Frankfurt–Munster group (Reiter et al, 1995) illustrates the good outcome for children with NHL. They treated 302 children, ≤ 18 years of age, with conventional chemo-radiotherapy for newly diagnosed NHL, including Burkitt's lymphoma (50%), lymphoblastic lymphoma (24%) and diffuse large-cell lymphomas, including Ki-1 (18%). The overall EFS for the whole group at 7 years was 80%. Thus, chemotherapy is the treatment of choice for NHL; however, for those patients who relapse, more intensive therapy is required to achieve a cure.

Stem cell transplantation using marrow or peripheral blood stem cells has a distinct advantage for relapsed NHL (DFS 18–62%) over continued conventional therapy where the DFS is at best 5–20% (Baro et al, 1991). Transplant outcome is dependent on several risk factors, including disease state at the time of transplant (remission versus active disease), failure to achieve a remission with initial therapy, LDH at the time of transplant, number of failed front line therapies, and clinical condition or performance status at the time of transplant (Gulati et al, 1988; Conde et al, 1994). Relapsed patients benefit from re-induction with conventional chemotherapy prior to transplant to reduce tumour burden.

There are few reports of bone marrow transplantation in NHL with only paediatric patients. In one report, four of five patients with relapsed diffuse large-cell NHL were re-induced with cytosine arabinoside, dexamethasone and cisplatin (DHAP) to achieve a second remission, and went on to ABMT, with all four disease-free a median of 3 years from transplant (Santana et al, 1993). One of the largest series reported children with relapsed or refractory NHL who received either autologous ($n = 23$) or allogeneic ($n = 1$), HLA matched sibling donor BMTs (Loiseau et al, 1991). Eight patients had lymphomas of T-cell origin, and sixteen had B-cell (Burkitt type) derived tumours. Prior to BMT, each patient (except one) was re-induced with secondary chemotherapy (etoposide, methotrexate, cisplatin, cytosine arabinoside) and nine were able to achieve a complete remission. The conditioning regimen for transplant included busulfan and either cyclophosphamide or melphalan or all three. Nineteen patients achieved a CR post-transplant, and eight patients (33%) survive disease free (7/16 B-cell and 1/8 T-cell) with a follow-up of 1–5 years. There are now several reports in the literature of using BMT successfully to treat relapsed Ki-1 lymphoma in children (Gordon et al, 1994) (Table 2). In a report from France (Troussard et al, 1990), seven of nine patients (five were ≤21 years old) with high-risk Burkitt's lymphoma survive after receiving HLA matched allogeneic transplants in first CR using TBI and cyclophosphamide as a preparative regimen.

Table 2. Bone marrow transplantation for non-Hodgkin's lymphoma.

Reference	Number of patients[1]	Treatment regimen[2]	DFS[3]/Follow-up
Gulati et al, 1988	31 (ABMT)	TBI + CY	48%/4 years
Petersen et al, 1990	101 (ABMT)	Bu/CY(12)	21%/5 years
Weaver et al, 1993		TBI + chemo (89)	
Weisdorf et al, 1991	70 (ABMT)	TBI + CY (57)	23%/3 years
		CY + BCNU + Ara-C (13)	
Baro et al, 1991	18 (ABMT)	TBI + CY	65%/3 years
Loiseau et al, 1991	24	BU ± CY ± melphalan	33%/3 years
	23 (ABMT), 1 (Allo)		
Chopra et al, 1992	938 (ABMT)	TBI or chemotherapy based	46%/40 months
	122 (Allo)		49%/48 months
Vose et al, 1993	158	TBI or chemotherapy based	29%/3 years
	105 (ABMT)		23%/3 years
	53 (PSCT)		40%/3 years
	Low risk features		45%/3 years
	High risk features		10%/3 years
Shepherd et al, 1993	21 (Allo)	TBI or chemotherapy based	38%/3 years
Conde et al, 1994	104 (ABMT)	TBI + CY (64)	51%/2 years
		chemotherapy based (40)	
Gordon et al, 1994	12	TBI + thiotepa ± VP-16	83%/32 months
	3 (Allo) + 9 (ABMT)		

[1] ABMT, autologous bone marrow transplant; Allo, allogeneic bone marrow transplant; PSCT, peripheral blood stem cell transplant.
[2] CY, cyclophosphamide; TBI, total body irradiation; BU, busulfan; chemotherapy based, reflects multiple chemotherapeutic regimens.
[3] DFS, disease free survival.

Because relatively few paediatric lymphomas go on to transplant, children are usually treated on adult protocols given their overall response is similar. The European Transplant Registry Group (Chopra et al, 1992) recently reviewed 1060 NHL cases and compared allogeneic and autologous BMT in case-matched patients. Children (age < 15 years) receiving allogeneic BMTs ($n = 17$) had a 38% progression-free survival after 48 months, while autologous grafts ($n = 17$) had a 40% progression-free survival after a median of 30 months. These results were not significantly different from the adults in the series. A lower relapse rate was found in the allogeneic group but at a cost of a higher transplant-related morbidity/mortality. Depending on patient selection and protocol enrollment, other studies in the literature have cited EFS of 10–83%, with 15–30% of patients in each series ≤21 years of age (Table 2). Autologous peripheral blood stem cells provide an additional source of stem cells if there is marrow involvement with lymphoma and early results appear to be as good as, or better than, autologous marrow transplantation.

SECOND TRANSPLANTS

Patients who have relapse of their leukaemia or lymphoma following transplantation have an extremely poor outcome, and because of their inability to tolerate additional chemotherapy, typically survive only short periods of time after relapse. Second marrow transplants have been attempted with 10–50% of patients surviving a median of 20 months (Barrett et al, 1985; Champlin et al 1985). Wagner et al (1992) reported second marrow transplants in 23 children and adults (median age, 29 years) with relapsed leukaemia following initial marrow transplant. A variety of conditioning regimens were used, and all patients received marrow grafts from the same donor with a median time between first and second transplants of 22.7 months. At 24 months post-second-transplant, the event-free survival was reported to be 38%, with the best outcome in patients with CML (7/12 survive). Thirty-five per cent of patients died by day 100 post-transplant, most commonly of relapsed disease (42% probability of relapse at 4–9 years).

Radich et al (1993) reported 77 adult and paediatric patients with leukaemia and lymphoma who had relapsed following allogeneic marrow transplants that utilized total-body irradiation and high-dose chemotherapy. The median time between transplants was 28 months. Preparative regimens for the second transplant included busulfan and cyclophosphamide or carmustine and etoposide. The DFS rate at 36 months was 14% overall with DFS of 8% for patients with ALL, 10% for AML, and 25% for CML with an overall probability of relapse of 70%. Veno-occlusive disease of the liver was the most frequent cause of transplant-related toxicity, with a day 100 nonrelapse mortality rate of 36%. Multivariate analysis demonstrated that the probability of DFS was associated with the presence of acute GVHD and age less than 10 years. Taken together, these studies suggest that some patients, particularly those with CML, and especially children, may benefit from a second marrow transplant following relapse of their leukaemia after initial transplantation.

FUTURE DIRECTIONS

Despite the encouraging results for high-dose chemoradiation therapy and bone marrow rescue for the treatment of children with leukaemia and lymphoma, only a minority of children will have a suitably matched related donor. Mismatched related marrow and unrelated donor marrow transplants are transplant options but at the cost of increased morbidity and mortality. Autologous marrow grafts are potentially complicated by the presence of residual tumour cells. The International Cord Blood Transplant Registry has reported 51 children, including 30 with malignant disease and 21 with non-malignant disease, who have received cord blood transplants from matched and mismatched donors who were both related and unrelated to the patient (Wagner et al, 1994). Interestingly, graft-versus-host disease has been minimal, despite marked HLA disparity in some of the transplants, suggesting that the use of cord blood stem cells may allow for transplantation across greater HLA barriers. Peripheral blood stem cells have been demonstrated to reconstitute haematopoiesis following myeloablative therapy for the treatment of malignant diseases (To et al, 1992). There are currently major research studies in progress investigating the use of peripheral blood stem cells from autologous and allogeneic sources.

The most significant barrier to successful stem cell transplantation remains the recurrence of malignant disease post-transplant. One approach being investigated to address this difficult problem involves the use of cytokines, including interleukin-2 and alpha-interferon, to modulate the immune system following transplantation in an attempt to generate or facilitate a graft-versus-leukaemia/lymphoma effect (Klingemann and Phillips, 1991). A second approach to enhance tumour kill involves increasing the amount of radiation delivered to malignant tissue prior to myeloablative doses of chemotherapy and radiation by selectively targeting leukaemia and lymphoma cells with monoclonal antibodies that are labelled with radioisotopes (Matthews et al, 1995). This innovative approach holds promise for intensifying therapy to malignant haematopoietic cells without increasing toxicity to normal tissues.

SUMMARY

Bone marrow transplantation has played a central and significant role in the successful treatment of childhood leukaemia and lymphoma. Bone marrow transplantation has expanded from a salvage therapy for children with relapsed disease to its current use as a front-line therapy for children with high-risk ALL, AML in 1st CR, and is currently the only known curative therapy for children with CML and JCML. Transplant in first relapse of HD or NHL has a clear advantage over transplantation after failure of multiple chemotherapy regimens. Advances in supportive care have decreased the toxicities attendant with the use of high-dose chemotherapy and irradiation followed by bone marrow rescue. The continued investigation and use of alternate sources of stem cells, as well as the development of better methods to kill tumour cells, will make this potentially curative form of therapy available to increasingly large number of children.

REFERENCES

Amadori S, Testi AM, Arico M et al (1993) Prospective comparative study of bone marrow transplantation and post-remission chemotherapy for childhood acute myelogenous leukaemia. *Journal of Clinical Oncology* **11:** 1046–1054.

Anderson JE, Litzow MR, Appelbaum FR et al (1993) Allogeneic, syngeneic, and autologous marrow transplantation for Hodgkin's disease: the 21 year Seattle experience. *Journal of Clinical Oncology* **11:** 2342–2350.

Armitage JO, Bierman PJ, Vose JM et al (1991) Autologous bone marrow transplantation for patients with relapsed Hodgkin's disease. *American Journal of Medicine* **91:** 605–611.

Barnett MJ, Eaves CJ, Phillips GL et al (1989) Successful autografting in chronic myeloid leukaemia after maintenance of marrow in culture. *Bone Marrow Transplantation* **12:** 345–351.

Baro J, Richard C, Calavia J et al (1991) Autologous bone marrow transplantation as consolidation therapy for non-Hodgkin's lymphoma patients with poor prognostic features. *Bone Marrow Transplantation* **8:** 283–289.

Barrett AJ, Tew C, Joshi R et al (1985) How should acute lymphoblastic leukaemia relapsing after bone-marrow transplantation be treated? *Lancet* **i:** 1188–1191.

Barrett AJ, Horowitz MM & Ash RC (1992) Bone marrow transplantation for Philadelphia chromosome-positive acute lymphoblastic leukaemia. *Blood* **79:** 3067–3070.

Barrett AJ, Horowitz MM & Pollock BH (1994) Bone marrow transplantation from HLA-identical siblings as compared with chemotherapy for children with acute lymphoblastic leukaemia in a second remission. *New England Journal of Medicine* **331:** 1253–1258.

Beatty PG, Ash R, Hows JM et al (1989) The use of unrelated bone marrow donors in the treatment of patients with chronic myelogenous leukaemia: experience of four marrow transplant centers. *Bone Marrow Transplantation* **4:** 287–290.

Bierman PJ, Vose JM & Armitage JO (1994) Autologous transplantation for Hodgkin's disease: coming of age. *Blood* **83:** 1161–1164.

Billet AL, Kornmehl E, Tarbell NJ et al (1993) Autologous bone marrow transplantation after a long first remission for children with recurrent acute lymphoblastic leukaemia. *Blood* **81:** 1651–1657.

Brenner MK, Rill DR, Moen RC et al (1993) Gene-marking to trace origin of relapse after autologous bone-marrow transplantation. *Lancet* **341:** 85–86.

Brochstein JA, Kernan NA, Groshen S et al (1987) Allogeneic bone marrow transplantation after hyperfractionated total-body irradiation and cyclophosphamide in children with acute leukaemia. *New England Journal of Medicine* **317:** 1618–1624.

Carella A, Podesta M, Frassoni F et al (1993) Selective overshoot of pH-negative blood hemopoietic cells after intensive idarubicin-containing regimen and their repopulating capacity after reinfusion. *Stem Cells* **11:** 67–72.

Castleberry RP, Emanuel PD, Zuckerman KS et al (1994) A pilot study of isotretinoin in the treatment of juvenile chronic myelogenous leukaemia. *New England Journal of Medicine* **331:** 1680–1684.

Champlin RE, Ho WG, Lenarsky C et al. (1985) Successful second bone marrow transplants for treatment of acute myelogenous leukaemia or acute lymphoblastic leukaemia. *Transplantation Proceedings* **17:** 496–499.

Chan HSL, Estrov Z, Weitzmann SS & Freedman MH (1987) The value of intensive combination chemotherapy for juvenile chronic myelogenous leukaemia. *Journal of Clinical Oncology* **5:** 1960–1967.

Chopra R, Goldstone AH, Pearce R et al (1992) Autologous versus allogeneic bone marrow transplantation for non-Hodgkin's lymphoma: a case controlled analysis of the European Bone Marrow Transplant Group Registry data. *Journal of Clinical Oncology* **10:** 1690–1695.

Chopra R, McMillan AK, Linch DC et al (1993) The place of high-dose BEAM therapy and autologous bone marrow transplantation in poor risk Hodgkin's disease: a single center eight year study of 155 patients. *Blood* **81:** 1137–1145.

Clift RA, Buckner CD, Thomas ED et al (1987) The treatment of acute non-lymphoblastic leukaemia by allogeneic marrow transplantation. *Bone Marrow Transplantation* **2:** 243–258.

Conde E, Sierra J, Iriondo A et al (1994) Prognostic factors in patients who received autologous bone marrow transplantation for non-Hodgkin's lymphoma. Report of 104 patients from the Spanish Cooperative Group GEL/TAMO. *Bone Marrow Transplantation* **14:** 279–286.

Coulombel L, Kalousek DK, Eaves CJ et al (1983) Long-term marrow culture reveals chromosomally normal hematopoietic progenitor cells in patients with Philadelphia chromosome-positive chronic myelogenous leukaemia. *New England Journal of Medicine* **308:** 1493–1498.

Creutzig UV, Ritter J, Schellong G et al (1990) Identification of two risk groups in childhood acute myelogenous leukaemia after therapy intensification in study AML-BFM-83 as compared with AML-BFM-78. *Blood* **75:** 1932–1941.

Creutzig U, Ritter J, Zimmerman M & Schellong G. (1993) Does cranial irradiation reduce the risk for bone marrow relapse in acute myelogenous leukaemia? Unexpected results of the childhood acute myelogenous leukaemia study BFM-87. *Journal of Clinical Oncology* **11:** 279–286.

Crump M, Smith AM, Brarndwein J et al (1993) High-dose etoposide and melphalan, and autologous bone marrow transplantation for patients with advanced Hodgkin's disease: importance of disease status at transplant. *Journal of Clinical Oncology* **11:** 704–711.

Deisseroth AB, Zu Z, Claxton D et al (1994) Genetic marking shows that pH+ cells present in autologous transplants of chronic myelogenous leukaemia contribute to relapse after autologous bone marrow in CML. *Blood* **83:** 3068–3076.

Forman SJ, Schmidt GM, Nademanee AP et al (1991) Allogeneic bone marrow transplantation as therapy for primary induction failure for patients with acute leukaemia. *Journal of Clinical Oncology* **9:** 1570–1574.

Fuchs R, Loffler M, Pfreundschuh M et al (1994) Prognosis of high dose chemotherapy/autologous bone marrow transplantation candidates not receiving this treatment after failure of primary therapy of Hodgkin's disease. *Leukaemia and Lymphoma* **14:** 79–89.

Gamis AS, Haake R, McGlave P & Ramsay NK (1993) Unrelated-donor bone marrow transplantation for Philadelphia chromosome-positive chronic myelogenous leukaemia in children. *Journal of Clinical Oncology* **11:** 834–838.

Gordon BG, Weisenburger DD, Sanger WG et al (1994) Peripheral T-cell lymphoma in children and adolescents: role of bone marrow transplantation. *Leukaemia and Lymphoma* **14:** 1–10.

Gorin NC, Najman A & Duhamel G (1977) Autologous bone marrow transplantation in acute myelocytic leukaemia. *Lancet* **i:** 1050.

Graham-Pole J (1989) Treating acute lymphoblastic leukaemia after relapse: bone marrow transplantation or not? *Lancet* **ii:** 1517.

Gulati SC, Shank B, Black P et al (1988) Autologous bone marrow transplantation for patients with poor-prognosis lymphoma. *Journal of Clinical Oncology* **6:** 1303–1313.

Haas R, Hohaus S, Egerer S et al (1992) Autologous blood stem cells transplantation in relapsed Hodgkin's disease. *International Journal of Cell Cloning* **10 (supplement 1):** 138–140.

Haines ME, Goldman JM, Worsley AM et al (1984) Chemotherapy and autografting for patients with chronic granulocytic leukaemia in transformation: probable prolongation of life for some patients. *British Journal of Haematology* **58:** 711–722.

Henze G, Fenger R, Hartmann R et al (1991) Six-year experience with a comprehensive approach to the treatment of recurrent childhood acute lymphoblastic leukaemia (ALL-REZ BFM 85): a relapse study of the BFM group. *Blood* **78:** 1166–1172.

Hunger SP, Link MP & Donaldson SS (1994) ABVD/MOPP and low-dose involved-field radiotherapy in pediatric Hodgkin's disease: the Stanford experience. *Journal of Clinical Oncology* **12:** 2160–2166.

Jones RJ, Ambinder RF, Piantadosi S et al (1991) Evidence of a graft-versus-lymphoma effect associated with allogeneic bone marrow transplantation. *Blood* **77:** 649–653.

Kantarjian HM, Deisseroth A, Kurzrock R et al (1993) Chronic myelogenous leukaemia: a concise update. *Blood* **82:** 691–703.

Kersey JH, Weisdorf D, Nesbit ME et al (1987) Comparison of autologous and allogeneic bone marrow transplantation for treatment of high-risk refractory acute lymphoblastic leukaemia. *New England Journal of Medicine* **317:** 461–467.

Kessinger A, Vose JM, Bierman PJ & Armitage JO (1992) High dose cyclophosphamide, etoposide, and carmustine and peripheral stem cell transplantation for patients with relapsed Hodgkin's disease and bone marrow abnormalities. *International Journal of Cell Cloning* **10 (supplement 1):** 135–137.

Klingebiel T, Creutzig U, Dopfer R et al (1990) Bone marrow transplantation in comparison with conventional therapy in children with adult type chronic myelogenous leukaemia. *Bone Marrow Transplantation* **5:** 317–320.

Klingemann H-G & Phillips GL (1991) Immunotherapy after bone marrow transplantation. *Bone Marrow Transplantation* **8:** 73–81.

Linch DC, Winfield D, Goldstone AH et al (1993) Dose intensification with autologous bone marrow transplantation in relapsed and resistant Hodgkin's disease: result of a BNLI randomized trial. *Lancet* **341:** 1051–1054.

Loiseau HA, Hartmann O, Valteau D et al (1991) High-dose chemotherapy containing busulfan followed by bone marrow transplantation in 24 children with refractory or relapsed non-Hodgkin's lymphoma. *Bone Marrow Transplantation* **8:** 465–472.

McGlave P, Arthur D, Haake R et al (1987) Therapy of chronic myelogenous leukaemia with allogeneic bone marrow transplantation. *Journal of Clinical Oncology* **5:** 1033–1040.

McGlave PB, Beatty P, Ash R et al (1990) Therapy for chronic myelogenous leukaemia with unrelated donor bone marrow transplantation: results in 102 cases. *Blood* **75:** 1728–1732.

Matthews DC, Appelbaum FR, Eary JF et al (1995) Development of a marrow transplant regimen for acute leukaemia using targeted hematopoietic irradiation delivered by ^{131}I-labeled anti-CD45 antibody, combined with cyclophosphamide and total body irradiation. *Blood* **85:** 1122–1131.

Michel G, Gluckman E, Blaise D et al (1992) Improvement in outcome for children receiving allogeneic bone marrow transplantation in first remission of acute myeloid leukaemia: a report from the Groupe d'etude des Greffes de Moelle Osseuse. *Journal of Clinical Oncology* **10:** 1865–1869.

Nesbit ME, Buckley JD, Feig SA et al (1994) Chemotherapy for induction of remission of childhood acute myeloid leukaemia followed by marrow transplantation or multiagent chemotherapy: a report from the Childrens Cancer Group. *Journal of Clinical Oncology* **12:** 127–135.

Petersen FB, Appelbaum FR, Hill R et al (1990) Autologous marrow transplantation for malignant lymphoma: a report of 101 cases from Seattle. *Journal of Clinical Oncology* **8:** 638–647.

Pinkel D (1993) Bone marrow transplantation in children. *Journal of Pediatrics* **122:** 331–340.

Pui C-H & Crist WM (1994) Biology and treatment of acute lymphoblastic leukaemia. *Journal of Pediatrics* **124:** 491–503.

Radich JP, Sanders JE, Buckner CD et al (1993) Second allogeneic marrow transplantation for patients with recurrent leukaemia after initial transplant with total-body irradiation-containing regimens. *Journal of Clinical Oncology* **11:** 304–313.

Reece DE, Barnett MJ, Connors JM et al (1991) Intensive chemotherapy with cyclophosphamide, carmustine, and etoposide followed by autologous bone marrow transplantation for relapsed Hodgkin's disease. *Journal of Clinical Oncology* **9:** 1871–1879.

Reece DE, Connors JM, Spinelli JJ et al (1994) Intensive therapy with cyclophosphamide, carmustine, etoposide ± cisplatin, and autologous bone marrow transplantation for Hodgkin's disease in first relapse after combination chemotherapy. *Blood* **83:** 1193–1199.

Reiffers J Trouette RK Marit G (1991) Autologous blood stem cell transplantation for chronic granulocytic leukaemia in transformation: a report of 47 cases. *British Journal of Haematology* **77:** 339–345.

Reiffers J, Goldman J, Meloni G et al (1994) Autologous stem cell transplantation in chronic myelogenous leukemia: a retrospective amalysis of the European Group for Bone Marrow Transplantation. *Bone Marrow Transplantation* **14:** 407–410.

Reiter A, Schrappe M, Parwaresch R et al (1995) Non-Hodgkin's Lymphomas of childhood and adolescence: results of a treatment stratified for biologic subtypes and stage—a report of the Berlin–Frankfurt–Munster Group. *Journal of Clinical Oncology* **13:** 359–372.

Sadowitz PD, Smith SD, Shuster J et al (1993) Treatment of late bone marrow relapse in children with acute lymphoblastic leukaemia: a Pediatric Oncology Group study. *Blood* **81:** 602–609.

Sallan SE, Niemeyer CM, Billet AL et al (1989) Autologous bone marrow transplantation for acute lymphoblastic leukaemia. *Journal of Clinical Oncology* **7:** 1594–1601.

Sanders JB, Thomas ED, Buckner CD et al (1985) Marrow transplantation for children in first remission of acute nonlymphoblastic leukemia: an update. *Blood* **66:** 460–462.

Sanders JE, Thomas ED, Buckner CD & Doney K (1987) Marrow transplantation for children with acute lymphoblastic leukaemia in second remission. *Blood* **70:** 324–326.

Sanders JE, Buckner CD, Thomas ED et al (1988) Allogeneic marrow transplantation for children with juvenile chronic myelogenous leukaemia. *Blood* **71:** 1144–1146.

Santana V, Ambromowitch M, Snadlund JT et al (1993) MA COP-B Treatment in children and adolescents with advanced diffuse large-cell non-Hodgkin's disease. *Leukaemia* **7:** 187–191.

Santos GW (1992) Allogeneic and autologous bone marrow transplantation in AML. *Leukaemia* **6:** 102–103.

Shepherd JD, Barnett MJ, Connors JM et al (1993) Allogeneic bone marrow transplantation for poor-prognosis non-Hodgkin's lymphoma. *Bone Marrow Transplantation* **12:** 591–596.

Smith FO, Sanders JE, Gooley T et al (1994) Allogeneic marrow transplantation for children with juvenile chronic myelogenous leukaemia. *Blood* **84:** 2012.

Speck B, Bortin MM, Champlin et al (1985) Allogeneic bone marrow transplantation for chronic myelogenous leukaemia. *Lancet* **i:** 665–668.

Spinolo JA, Jagannath S, Velasquez W et al (1993) Cisplatin-CBV with autologous bone marrow transplantation for relapsed Hodgkin's disease. *Leukaemia and Lymphoma* **9:** 7–77.

Thomas ED & Clift RA (1989) Indications for marrow transplantation in chronic myelogenous leukaemia. *Blood* **73:** 861–864.

Thomas ED, Buckner CD, Banaji M et al (1977) One hundred patients with acute leukaemia treated by chemotherapy, total body irradiation, and allogeneic marrow transplantation. *Blood* **49:** 511–533.

Thomas ED, Clift RA, Fefer A, et al (1986) Marrow transplantation for the treatment of chronic myelogenous leukaemia. *Annals of Internal Medicine* **104:** 155–163.

Tiedemann K, Waters KD, Tauro GP et al (1993) Results of intensive therapy in childhood acute myeloid leukaemia, incorporating high-dose melphalan and autologous bone marrow transplantation in first complete remission. *Blood* **82:** 3730–3738.

To LB, Roberts MM & Haylock DN (1992) Comparison of haematological recovery times and supportive care requirements of autologous recovery phase peripheral blood stem cell transplants, autologous bone marrow transplants and allogeneic bone marrow transplants. *Bone Marrow Transplantation* **9:** 277–284.

Tourani JM, Levy R, Colonna P et al (1992) High-dose salvage chemotherapy without bone marrow transplantation for adult patients with refractory Hodgkin's disease. *Journal of Clinical Oncology* **10:** 1086–1094.

Troussard X, Leblong V, Kuentz M et al (1990) Allogeneic bone marrow transplantation in adults with Burkitt's lymphoma or acute lymphoblastic leukaemia in first complete remission. *Journal of Clinical Oncology* **10:** 1086–1094.

Vose JM, Anderson JR, Kessinger A et al (1993) High-dose chemotherapy and autologous hematopoietic stem-cell transplantation for aggressive non-Hodgkin's lymphoma. *Journal of Clinical Oncology* **11:** 1846–1851.

Wagner JE, Vogelsang GB, Zehnbauer BA et al (1992) Relapse of leukaemia after bone marrow transplantation: effect of second myeloablative therapy. *Bone Marrow Transplantation* **9:** 205–209.

Wagner JE, Kernan NA, Broxmeyer HE & Gluckman E (1994) Transplantation of umbilical cord blood in 50 patients: analysis of the registry data. *Blood* **84:** 395a.

Weaver CH, Appelbaum FR, Petersen FB et al (1993) Follow-up report on the outcome of patients relapsing after autologous marrow transplantation for malignant lymphoma. *Journal of Clinical Oncology* **11:** 812–813.

Weisdorf DJ, Haake R, Miller WJ et al (1991) Autologous bone marrow transplantation for progressive non-Hodgkin's lymphoma: clinical impact of immunophenotype and *in vitro* purging. *Bone Marrow Transplantation* **8:** 135–142.

Wells RJ, Woods WG, Buckley JD et al (1994) Treatment of newly diagnosed children and adolescents with acute myeloid leukaemia: a Children's Cancer Group study. *Journal of Clinical Oncology* **12:** 2367–2377.

Williams CD, Goldstone AH, Pearce R et al (1993) Autologous bone marrow transplantation for pediatric Hodgkin's disease: a case-matched comparison with adult patients by the European Bone Marrow Transplant Group Lymphoma Registry. *Journal of Clinical Oncology* **11:** 2243–2249.

Woods WG, Kobrinsky N, Buckley J et al (1993) Intensively timed induction therapy followed by autologous or allogeneic bone marrow transplantation for children with acute myeloid leukaemia or myelodysplastic syndrome: a Children's Cancer Group pilot study. *Journal of Clinical Oncology* **11:** 1448–1457.

Yahalom J, Gulati SC, Toia M et al (1993) Accelerated hyperfractionated totallymphoid irradiation, high-dose chemotherapy, and autologous bone marrow transplantation for refractory and relapsing patients with Hodgkin's disease. *Journal of Clinical Oncology* **11:** 1062–1070.

Zander AR, Dicke KA, Keating M et al (1985) Allogeneic bone marrow transplantation for acute leukaemia refractory to induction chemotherapy. *Cancer* **56:** 1374–1379.

7

Treatment of acute myeloid leukaemia in children

SVERRE O. LIE

The progress in the treatment of childhood malignancies is well known and well documented. However, we are still very far from curing every child with such a diagnosis. In 1992, almost twice as many children died of cancer than of traffic accidents in Norway.

This chapter will focus on the therapy of acute myelogenous leukaemia (AML) in children. In an article on childhood cancer survival in the USA during 1973–87, AML was announced as the 'childhood tumor with the most dismal prognosis' (Novakovic, 1994). It is certainly a much more complex and resistant disease than the lymphoblastic variant (ALL), although progress in recent years has given event-free survivals of between 20 and 40% in many major multicentre studies.

Although the major focus of this chapter will be on therapy, a brief review of epidemiology and pathogenesis will be given as a background. The main emphasis will be on publications from the last 3–4 years. For developments before 1989, the reader is referred to some recent comprehensive reviews (Lie, 1989; Boulad and Kernan, 1993; Ravindranath and Schultz, 1994). Naturally, examples will also be drawn from the experiences of the Nordic Society for Paediatric Haematology and Oncology (NOPHO) which has run a population-based registry of all childhood leukaemias since 1981 and has had common protocols for AMLs since 1984 (Lie and Gustafsson, 1992).

EPIDEMIOLOGY

In the Nordic countries, the incidence of all acute leukaemias is 4.6 new cases per year per 100 000 children younger than 15 years of age (Table 1). The majority are, of course, ALL, while AML develops in slightly fewer than 1 child per 100 000 per year and accounts for 17% of all acute leukaemias. As can be seen from the table, the incidence is very similar in the five Nordic countries. In the United States there are approximately 350 new cases of childhood AML per year (Boulad and Kernan, 1993), while 1258 new cases were reported in Great Britain in the period 1971–88 (Stiller and Eatock, 1994). The ratio of boys to girls in our series is about

Baillière's Clinical Paediatrics—
Vol. 3, No. 4, November 1995
ISBN 0–7020–2075–3

Table 1. Annual incidence of acute childhood leukaemias in the Nordic countries (1984–92).

	All acute leukaemias*	AML*
Denmark	4.6	0.8
Finland	4.8	0.6
Iceland	4.1	0.9
Norway	4.2	0.8
Sweden	4.7	0.8
Total	4.6	0.7

* Per 100 000 children less than 15 years of age.

1:1, which is in contrast to most other publications where the ratio of boys to girls is approximately 1.3 to 1. In black children the relative incidence of AML is significantly higher due to a lower incidence of ALL.

We have seen a definite peak incidence in the younger age group which has not been seen in other series (Neglia and Robison, 1988). One explanation could be the high frequency of children with Down syndrome (DS) in our series (Slørdahl et al, 1993). Children with trisomy 21 actually account for 13% of all new cases and have a much younger age at diagnosis than normal children. In the big German and Italian studies, children with DS are not mentioned, which means that they are probably not included (Creutzig et al, 1990, 1993; Amadori et al, 1993). In the UK, 5.1% of children with AML are reported to be DS (Stiller and Eatock, 1994), while a big survey conducted by the Children's Cancer Group (CCG) in the USA reported 2% of the AML cases to be DS (Robison et al, 1984). In a Paediatric Oncology Group study, 12 of 285 children (4%) had DS (Ravindranath et al, 1992).

The aetiology remains unknown in the vast majority of cases. However, some genetic diseases and environmental factors have been implicated as predisposing factors in some children. It has been shown that the risk of leukaemia is increased in an identical twin of a child with AML, but is not significantly higher in non-twin siblings. Among genetic diseases with a predisposition to leukaemia (besides the Down syndrome) are chromosomal instabilities like Bloom's syndrome, Fanconis anaemia and ataxia telangiectasia. Studies on environmental factors have focused both on exposures in utero and postnatally. The CCG has run a case–control study of 204 patients and shown that paternal or maternal exposure to pesticides and petroleum products increases the risk of leukaemia in their offspring. A very significant risk was associated with the maternal use of marihuana (Neglia and Robison, 1988). Environmental factors, such as high doses of ionizing irradiation, are well known.

In recent years particular attention has been paid to the development of secondary AML seen after agressive chemotherapy. The risk of AML after Hodgkin's disease is well documented and often shows chromosomal abnormalities involving numbers 5 and 7 which have a FAB-type M1/M2. A most disturbing relationship has recently been found between the use of epipodophyllotoxins and secondary AML. A recent review estimated that children with ALL treated with high doses of epipodophyllotoxins (VP-16 and/or VM-26) have a cumulative risk of 5–12% of developing a secondary AML (Winick et al, 1993; Sugita et al, 1993; Smith et al, 1994a). This AML is different from that seen after alkylating agents in that there is a shorter latency period and the majority of cases involve changes in chromosome 11q23 and are of FAB type M4/M5. Myelodysplasia and secondary AML are also increasingly seen in patients receiving myeloablative therapy with autologous stem-cell transplantation. Actuarial risks as high as 18% ±9% have recently been reported (reviewed by Rohatiner, 1994). Certainly, if these bone marrow 'lethal' therapies are going to increase in number, this is a problem of increasing concern.

BIOLOGY

In order to understand the pathogenesis of AML it is necessary to understand the present concept of normal haemopoiesis. It is widely accepted that all haemopoietic cells, including lymphocytes, orginate from a common multipotent stem cell and that the haemopoietic system can be divided into several compartments in a hierarchy of development. The mature cells seen in peripheral blood—such as erythrocytes, polymorphonuclear granulocytes, monocytes and platelets—arise from bone marrow progenitors that are committed to differentiation along a single lineage. These committed stem cells have limited proliferative capabilites and are supposed to give rise to only a limited class of peripheral blood cells. Their names and their growth factors are derived from in vitro techniques, where such committed stem cells give rise to distinct colonies when plated in soft agar with the appropriate growth factors present. The colony forming unit (CFU) of granulocytes (G) requires granulocyte colony stimulating factor (G-CSF) for growth in vitro. The other committed stem cells are CFU-GM (granulocyte and macrophages) which require GM-CSF for growth, CFU-M (macrophages) which require M-CSF (or CSF-1) for growth, and CFU-erythroid which requires erythropoietin for growth. These four growth factors (cytokines) (G-CSF, GM-CSF, M-CSF and erythropoietin) are available in recombinant form, and their genes have been cloned and localized. Recently, the stem cell factor (c-kit ligand) and thrombopoietin (M pl ligand) have also been characterized (reviewed by Metcalf, 1994a,b).

It should be emphasized that these cytokines act in a complex interplay and that other signals such as the various interleukins (IL-3, IL-6) and interferons also participate in the regulation of blood cell synthesis.

The committed progenitors are derived from the pluripotent (multilineage) haemopoietic stem cells (CFU-mix) that give rise to new haemopoietic stem cells ('birth') or generate primitive but committed progenitors ('death'). Lymphocytes are thought to be generated from these cells and to form progenitors with more extensive self-renewal capabilities. They will not be discussed further.

It is clear that the majority of cases of AML are of a monoclonal (unicellular) origin representing cells with a mutational event at some stage in their early development. The malignant cell retains the capacity of self renewal, but not of maturation. Our classification of the leukaemias depends on where in the normal haemopoietic development the mutation has taken place, and using immunological, enzymatic and molecular probes it is possible to establish the cell lineage in most cases.

The modified French–American–British (FAB) classifications from 1985 distinguished between seven distinct subgroups (M1–M7) on the basis of conventional morphology, cytochemical and immunological methods (Bennett et al, 1985). Recently M0 has been defined by the same working group as a very undifferentiated leukaemia (Bennett et al, 1991). The characteristic features of each FAB group is given in Table 2.

Table 2. FAB classification and childhood AML.

FAB class	Histochemistry*	Cell-surface markers	Associated cytogenetic findings
M1	MP+	CD33+, CD13+, CD11+ HLA DR+	+8, −5, −7
M2	MP+	CD33+, CD13+, CD11+	t(8;21)
M3	MP+	CD33+, CD13+, CD11+	t(15;17)
M4	MP+ NSE+	CD33+, CD13+, CD11+ HLA DR+	inv 16
M5	NSE+	CD33+, CD13+, CD11+ HLA DR +	t(1;11) t(9;11)
M6	PAS+ MP+	Glycophorine + spectrin + HLA DR+	
M7	PPO+	Glycoprotein IIb/IIIa (CD 41) or IIIa (CD 61)+	inv 3 or t(3;3), t(1;23)
M8	MP− NSF−	CD33+, CD13+, CD14+ HLA DR−	

* MP = myeloperoxidase; NSE = non-specific esterase; PPO = platelet peroxidase.
(Modified from Ravindranath and Schultz, 1994.)

M0 and M1 are sometimes difficult to distinguish from a leukaemia in the lymphoid lineage. We have found immunophenotypic classification to be most helpful in addition to conventional histochemistry (Ludwig et al, 1994). The specific myeloid markers include CD13 (cluster of differentiation), CD14 and CD33. The presence of B-cell markers (CD10, CD19, CD20) and/or T-cell markers (CD2, CD3, CD7) can occasionally be detected in a small concentration on myeloid leukaemic cells, but should not be present in large numbers. If the leukaemic cell at the same time expresses both myeloid and lymphoid antigens, the leukaemia is considered to be biphenotypic. In rare instances, we can also find that different malignant cells express, independently, myeloid and lymphoid markers, and the leukaemia is then considered to be bilineal. The origin of these hybrid leukemias is unclear. The possible impact of the presence or absence of specific markers and prognosis is still unclear.

Table 3 shows the distribution of FAB-types in seven large studies, including 1471 children. The distribution is rather similar with slightly less than half of the cases being M1/M2, c. 10% M3, 20–25% M4, about 20% M5, and 10% M6/M7.

Table 3. Percentage of children with different FAB subtypes.

	UK[a]	BFM-83[b]	BFM-87[b]	AIEOP[c]	CCG 2861[d]	NOPHO 84/88[e]	POG 8498[f]
M0, undifferentiated	–	–	4	–	–	–	–
M1, myeloblastic undifferentiated	10	20	12	12	10	20	47 (M1 and M2)
M2, myeloblastic differentiated	20	20	27	27	26	27	
M3, promyelocytic	6	3	5	17	11	6	3
M4, myelomonocytic	23	25	25	16	24	16	27
M5, monoblastic	12	26	23	18	17	14	14
M6, erythroblastic	4	4	3	10 (M6 and M7)	3	5	1
M7, megakaryoblastic	6	2	4		8.5	3	3
Unknown	19	–	4	?	–	9	5
Number of children	283	182	210	161	129	221	285

[a] Stiller and Eatock (1994).
[b] Creutzig et al (1993).
[c] Amadori et al (1993).
[d] Wells et al (1994).
[e] Unpublished.
[f] Ravindranath et al (1991).

Progress in cytogenetics has confirmed the value of the FAB classification in that specific chromosomal translocations can be assigned to each group. Translocation between chromosome 8 and 21 [t(8;21)] is found almost exclusively in M1 and M2. All cases of M3 should carry the translocation t(15;17), and M5 is associated with t(9;11). Finally, abnormalities of chromosome 16 are seen predominantly in M4 and are often associated with increased eosinophils in the marrow.

In infants, chromosomal changes involving 11q23 are very common (Chen et al, 1993; Thirman et al, 1993). Many different chromosomes can participate in translocations involving this locus (Gu et al, 1992). The gene on chromosome 11 which is involved (called MLL, HRX or ALL-1) has recently been characterized and it turns out to be closely related to a homeobox gene in *Drosophila* which, when mutated, gives rise to bizarre morphological malformations of the thorax and abdomen in these organisms.

Other gene products of the specific translocations have recently been identified (Cline, 1994). In t(15;17) translocation seen in the promyelocytic leukaemias (FAB M3), the break point on chromosome 17 is in a gene encoding the retinoic acid nuclear receptor alpha (RAR-α) and on chromosome 15 in a gene initially called *myl* and later renamed PML (see review by Warrell et al, 1993). It is one of the most exciting developments in the biology of leukaemias that this leukaemia is responding to all-trans retinoic acid.

The gene product of the t(8;21) (q22;q22) translocation has also been detected recently. The chromosomal breakpoint on chromosome 21 involves a gene called AML-1 and the probable candidate on chromosome 8 is a gene called EOT. As usual, this translocation results in the production of a chimeric gene and a message that eventually may lead to a malignancy (Downing et al, 1993; Maseki et al, 1993; Nucifora et al, 1993).

The tumour suppressor gene WT1, which is implicated in the development of some cases of Wilms' tumour, has recently been shown to be detectable in all of 45 patients with AML examined (Inoue et al, 1994) and it seems that high expression is associated with a poor prognosis. The role of the tumour-suppressor gene p53 has recently been reviewed (Imamura et al, 1994).

Clinical presentation

Although AML is certainly a more complex disease than ALL, the clinical presentation might be indistinguishable. Lack of normal mature blood cells may result in anaemia, bleeding and infections. More than 50% have hepatosplenomegaly, while adenopathy is less frequent. The incidence of central nervous system involvement was present in only 9 of 221 (4%) cases in the Nordic material. Usually the CNS involvement is clinically silent. Chloromas (also called granulocytic sarcoma) are localized collections of leukaemic cells seen almost exclusively in patients with AML. These may occur at any site, including CNS, bone and skin, and even orbital chloromas can be seen.

It should be emphasized that AML may present as an acute emergency with life-threathening complications such as infections, haemorrhage or organ dysfunction secondary to leukostasis. In the Nordic material 3 out of the first 292 patients died before any therapy could be instituted.

Sometimes the diagnosis of leukaemia is preceeded by a prolonged preleukaemic phase lasting several weeks or months. Usually this is characterized by a lack of one of the normal blood cell lineages, resulting in either a refractory anaemia, a moderate degree of neutropenia or thrombocytopenia. Bone marrow examinations fail to detect a leukaemia, but there are definite morphological changes. This condition is often referred to as a myelodysplastic syndrome (MDS) which has its own FAB classification (Hasle, 1994). Usually it is a requirement that this diagnosis should have a hypercellular marrow, but in our experience this is not always the case. Some children may be seen with a hypoplastic marrow that later develops into an acute leukaemia.

THERAPY

Thirty years ago less than 5% of children with AML survived. Today, survival figures of more than 40% are reported in many studies, including the Nordic population-based material (for references, see Table 4). The change came in the beginning of the 1970s with the introduction of cytarabine (Ara-C) and anthracyclines. With different combinations of these drugs remission could be induced in about 75–85% of the children. However, without further therapy most children relapsed within a year. It became increasingly apparent that the resistance of the myeloblasts to therapy necessitated an intensity of therapy which certainly was on the border of what a child could tolerate. Death in aplasia and even death in complete remission have been the price we have had to pay for the progress we have seen. For every child going into a modern AML protocol, the morbidity is very significant, and life-threathening complications have to be dealt with. For example, in a series from Great Ormond Street (Phillips et al, 1991), two groups of patients where compared, diagnosed 1972–1982 ('modest' therapy) and 1983–1987 (intensive therapy). In the first group the median stay in hospital was 35 days, compared with 170 days in the latter group. As expected, this group received much more intravenous antibiotics and total parenteral nutrition. Modern therapy of AML is therefore justified only in larger centres, as the children often need complex support and must at times be monitored as an intensive care patient. In the Medical Research Council (MRC) AML trials in Great Britain it has been shown that children entered in national trials had a higher survival rate than those treated elsewhere, and that children treated at teaching hospitals had the best outcome (Stiller and Eatock, 1994). Needless to say, the availability of psychosocial care and the need to handle the patient and the whole familiy in an environment of total care is a prerequisite, although a topic outside the scope of this chapter.

Therapy is divided into several phases, all of which have as their aim the eradication of the malignant clone. During remission induction, the aggressive cytostatic therapy which is administered results in normal haematopoietic recovery and the disappearance of all leukaemic cells in those children who achieve remission. However, leukaemia will almost always return if therapy is stopped at this point. Intensive post-remission chemotherapy is therefore necessary; it is usually called consolidation or early intensification. Bone marrow transplantation (being autologous or allogeneic) is the most aggressive example of consolidation therapy. Maintenance therapy is generally viewed as multiple courses of less aggressive chemotherapy given over months or years.

Induction chemotherapy

In spite of the fact that AML is many different diseases, there is no significant evidence that different leukaemias need different approaches. One notable exception to this rule is promyelocytic leukaemia (M3) (see below). Table 4 presents the results of induction of some recently reported trials. For earlier studies the reader is referred to earlier reviews. For the most part, patients were recruited after 1984, except for the CCG-251 study which recruited patients from 1979–1983, but where the definitive manuscript was published in 1994.

Space does not allow a detailed description of the individual protocols. The drugs used are indicated in the table, but for details the reader must seek the original paper. With a variety of induction regimens, the remission rate was very close to 80% in all studies. The failures were due to resistant disease and death in aplasia.

Very few studies have compared different induction regimens in a prospective way. One exception is CCG-213 with 591 evaluable patients. In this study a standard induction regimen of Ara-C and daunorubicin ('7+3') was compared with a regimen containing these drugs ('5 + 2') plus VP-16, thioguanine and dexamethasone. The addition of the three extra drugs did not influence the induction rate, or the ultimate outcome.

Another question of importance is whether the intensity of the induction regimen has any impact on the eventual outcome. In the first Nordic study (NOPHO-84), death during aplasia was a minor problem compared with resistant disease (Table 4, Lie et al, 1990). In the 1984 protocol, induction therapy was of modest intensity and consisted of three series including Ara-C (100 mg/m^2 i.v. q12 h days 1, 2, 3, 4), 6-thioguanine (100 mg/m^2 p.o. q12 h days 1, 2, 3, 4), and doxorubicin (75 mg/m^2 day 5). The main reason for failure was resistant disease using this combination. Consequently, in our next study we added VP-16 and mitoxantrone to the induction regimen, with courses spaced as close together as possible. This resulted in an almost complete disappearance of resistant disease, but we had to pay the price since more children died in aplasia. The ultimate outcome has so far not been significantly different.

A most challenging preliminary report has been published where so called 'timed intensive induction therapy' has been compared with standard

Table 4. Results of induction chemotherapy in childhood AML.

	CCG-251[a]	CCG-213[b]	POG-8498[c]	CCG-2861[d]	AIEOP[e]	BFM-83[f]	BFM-87[f]	MRC-10[g]	NOPHO-84[h]	NOPHO-88[h]
Years entered	1979–83	1986–89	1984–88	1986–89	1987–90	1982–86	1986–91	1988–93	1984–88	1988–92
Number evaluable	490	591	285	142	161	173	210	270	105	118
Chemotherapy	Ara-C + Dauno ('7 + 3') or Ara-C + Doxo 2–4 courses	'7 + 3' or '5 + 2' + VP-16, Dexa, 6 TG	Dauno, Ara-C, 6TG (DAT) × 2 or DAT × 1 and high-dose Ara-C	Dexa Ara-C, 6-TG, VP-16, Dauno (DCTER)	'7 + 3' + '5 + 2'	Ara-C, Dauno, VP-16, Predn., 6-TG, VCR, Adr + Cytox		Ara-C, Dauno, VP-16 (ADE) versus Dauno, Ara-C, 6-TG (DAT)	Modified DAT	Modified DAT + VP-16, Mitox
Death in aplasia	50	38	19	19	6 (+6)	12	11	25 (death in aplasia and resistant disease)	8	14
Resistant disease	59	89	24	15	22	22	35		15	4
Complete remission	381 (78%)	439 (77%)	242 (85%)	108 (76%)	127 (79%)	139 (80%)	164 (78%)	245 (91%)	82 (78%)	100 (85%)

[a] Nesbit et al (1994).
[b] Wells et al (1994).
[c] Ravindranath et al (1991).
[d] Woods et al (1993).
[e] Amadori et al (1993).
[f] Creutzig et al (1993).
[g] Stevens et al (1994).
[h] Lie et al (1992).

timing (Woods et al, 1994). The very intensive 'timed induction' did not improve the percentage of children entering remission, but certainly improved the post-remission outcome. Among 382 patients, 60% treated in the intensive induction regimen remain disease-free, compared with only 37% in the standard induction arm ($P < 0.002$). The authors conclude that the timed intensive approach does not improve the remission rate, but markedly increased the long-term outcome regardless of the type of post-remission therapy utilized. Neither the recent experience of the UK MRC 10 trial nor the Nordic experience are in complete agreement with this view.

Post-remission therapy

Remission is far from cure. There has been one definite trend in post-remission therapy in recent years, and that has been to intensify. In many ways AML has long been the testing stone for the concept of dose intensity. Table 5 shows the result of post-remission therapy in the same studies outlined in Table 4. Different, but all very intensive protocols, have been explored of which the ultimate is bone marrow ablative therapy followed by an allogeneic or autologus transplant. Again, details of the protocols used in the various studies cannot be outlined due to lack of space, but the drugs used are indicated.

One of the most common approaches in post-remission therapy is to use high-dose Ara-C either alone or in combination with other agents. In our unit we introduced high-dose Ara-C in post-remission therapy of AML in 1982 and have presented our results earlier (Lie and Slørdahl, 1985). Our first Nordic study utilized high dose Ara-C (2 g/m^2 12 hours × 6) as the only post-remission therapy (Lie et al, 1990). The POG study 8498 also relied heavily on high-dose Ara-C as well as CCG and BFM in their most recent studies. However, no one has really been sure about the optimal way of using Ara-C after more than 20 years of use. One of the first really randomized studies on different doses was published in 1994 by Mayer et al. They randomized patients who had a complete remission to receive four courses of Ara-C at three different doses: 100 mg/m^2/day for 5 days versus 400 mg/m^2/day for 5 days versus 3 g/m^2 q 12 hours on days 1, 3 and 5. Their data supported the concept of a dose–response effect for Ara-C in patients with AML younger than 60 years of age. With the highest dose they achieved results comparable to those reported in patients who had undergone allogeneic bone marrow transplantation in first remission.

In a recent editorial, the concept of dose intensity has been thoroughly analysed by Berman (1995). He questions whether there really is any dose effect with anthracyclines but does acknowledge a dosage effect when it comes to Ara-C. However, he points out that the benefit is seen only in patients less than 60 years of age and in patients with favourable prognosis.

The role of bone marrow transplantation (BMT)

Allogeneic BMT using an HLA matched sibling donor is now an established therapy for many haematological malignancies. More than 5000

Table 5. Results of post-remission therapy in childhood AML.

	CCG-251[a]	CCG-213[b]	POG-8498[c]	CCG-2861[d]	AIEOP[e]	BFM-83[f]	BFM-87[f]	MRC-10[g]	NOPHO-84[h]	NOPHO-88[h]
Years entered	1979–83	1986–89	1984–88	1986–89	1987–90	1982–86	1986–91	1988–93	1984–88	1988–92
Complete remission (%)	78	77	85	76	79	80	78	91	78	85
Post-remission therapy	Allo BMT when donor or Maintenance: continuous versus cyclic	BMT versus high-dose Ara-C + asp (Capizzi) Maintenance: non versus 'PATCO'	High-dose Ara-C + asp, VP-16, Azac, predn., vincr., methotr., 6-MP, Ara-C	Allo versus auto BMT	DAT, Allo or auto BMT or maintenance	6 drugs predn, Doxo, cytox, vincr, Ara-C, 6-TG)	6 drugs (Predn, doxo, cytox, vincr, Ara-C, 6-TG) + late intensification (high dose Ara-C + VP-16	Allo versus Auto versus no further therapy	High-dose Ara-C	High dose Ara-C + Mitox, VP-16
pDFS (%)	40	39	45	40	31	61	52	56	43	56

[a] Nesbit et al (1994).
[b] Wells et al (1994).
[c] Ravindranath et al (1991).
[d] Woods et al (1993).
[e] Amadori et al (1993).
[f] Creutzig et al (1993).
[g] Stevens et al (1994).
[h] Lie et al (1992).

transplants are performed yearly world-wide (Giralt and Champlin, 1994) for a variety of conditions, of which the most accepted indications are chronic myelogenous leukaemia in a stable phase, immune deficiencies and some metabolic disorders. The role of allogeneic BMT in acute myelogenous leukaemia is still a matter of dispute. Table 6 shows some recent randomized studies where allogeneic BMT has been offered to all patients with an HLA-matched leukocyte-culture-negative sibling and where the results have been compared with those receiving an autologous graft or intensive chemotherapy only. It is unfortunate that from some abstracts it is difficult to get the actual number of patients in the autologous transplanted and 'chemotherapy-only' groups. Such numbers have therefore been deleted from the table. It is important to note that a matched transplant is an option for only about 20% of the children who enter complete remission. In the Nordic countries this option is even smaller due to low numbers of siblings.

Table 6. Bone marrow transplantation in childhood AML.

	Number in CR	Allo-BMT Number	Allo-BMT DFS (%)	Auto BMT DFS (%)	Chemotherapy only DFS (%)
CCG 251[a]	381	85	50	—	36
CCG 213[b]	439	92	46	—	38
CCG 2861[c]	108	16	55	51	—
MRC AML-10[d]	766	174	58	54	52
AIEOP/LAM 87[e]	127	22	51	21	27
Total	1821	389 (21%)			

[a] Nesbit et al (1994).
[b] Wells et al (1994).
[c] Woods et al (1993).
[d] Burnett et al (1994).
[e] Amadori et al (1993).

In the first randomized study (CCG 251) allogeneic transplant clearly gave a superior disease-free survival compared with a continuous or a cyclic maintenance regimen ($P<0.05$). However, in a later study from the same group (CCG 213) with more intensive induction and post-remission therapy, comparisions of BMT to chemotherapy favoured BMT, but the difference was too small to reach statistical significance (Wells et al, 1994). In their most recent study (Woods et al, 1994) it was the intensity of the *induction* regimen that was the variable with the greatest impact and there was no difference in disease-free survival between the transplantation and the chemotherapy group. In the big UK MRC-10 trial there is so far no difference between the allo-, autologous or intensive chemotherapy arms (Burnett et al, 1994).

In the literature there are numerous reports from single centres on the positive results of allo BMT in AML. The methods have created a lot of controversy and the main problem has been the problem of patient selection. Since bone marrow transplants are usually performed many months after entering remission, this group is difficult to compare with those children receiving chemotherapy alone, since many of them actually relapse before they have a chance to receive a bone marrow transplant. Therefore, more recent studies have analysed the data according to the 'intention-to-treat' principle, which means that patients with an HLA-matched sibling are compared to those without, regardless of whether they receive the transplant or not. This has been the method used in all studies mentioned in Table 6.

The scope of this chapter does not include the management of adults, but an important paper from a cooperative group in Europe has recently appeared (Zittoun et al, 1995). In a prospective study, three different post-remission therapies were compared in adult patients: intensive therapy ($n=126$), autologous BMT ($n=128$) and allogeneic BMT ($n=168$). Disease-free survival was significantly inferior in the arm receiving chemotherapy, although the difference in terms of survival was not significant. The higher incidence of early mortality after allogeneic transplantation was counter-balanced by a lower incidence of late mortality in that group. It is of interest to note that the conclusions of this impressive and prospective study were questioned in an editorial in the same journal (Löwenberg, 1995).

Because less than 20% of patients have an HLA identical donor, an increasing amount of effort has been invested in establishing registries of volunteer unrelated donors. Many of these are now associated in the World Marrow Donor Association (Goldman, 1994). The use of unrelated donors as post-remission therapy in AML is still experimental and should be performed only in a scientific setting. The morbidity is significant, and in a recent study 40% of unrelated recipients died in remission (Busca et al, 1994). Something resembling a 'brave new world' is opening up when we read about freezing stem cells of cord-blood for eventual use later in life (Gale, 1995).

Even after a bone marrow transplant, however, relapse of the underlying disease remains the most frequent cause of treatment failure in addition to transplant-related mortality. Relapse rates in recent reports range from 10 to 40% depending on patient selection, treatment regimen and length of follow up (Giralt and Champlin, 1994).

One specific morbidity of bone marrow transplant is graft-versus-host disease (GVHD). Using unrelated donors, this problem is even more important. GVHD is divided into an acute and a chronic form. This problem continues to be the major complication after allogeneic BMT, and the disease—and in particular the immunological mechanism behind the disease—has recently been reviewed by Vogelsang and Hess (1994). It is of interest that even self antigens may play a role in GVHD and that cytokines may play a more central role, mediating many of the clinical manifestations of GVHD in addition to the direct cytotoxicity mediated by the alloreactive T-cells. Certainly, the graft versus leukaemia effect has been well documented (Nesbit et al, 1994).

The high relapse rate in AML and the possible improvement in results when using allogeneic BMT as post-remission therapy have stimulated the development of autologous bone marrow transplant. In this technique the patient's bone marrow is harvested during remission and preserved in liquid nitrogen. Bone marrow ablative therapy is then given and the marrow is thawed and re-infused. The marrow may or may not be purged with drugs such as 4-hydroperoxy-cyclophosphamide (4-HC) or monoclonal antibodies in order to remove contaminating leukaemic cells.

As shown in Table 6, this modality of therapy is also very difficult to evaluate. Different studies are difficult to compare, but many prospective randomized studies are underway. What has been obvious during the last year is that the larger prospective studies which have addressed this question have so far not been able to show any significant benefit of autologous bone marrow transplant in childhood AML. The main reason for this is probably that the increased intensity of chemotherapy alone has improved outcome so that the benefit of transplantation is much more difficult to detect.

Both for allogeneic and autologous bone marrow transplant the use of peripheral stem cells has attracted great interest in recent years. The peripheral haemopoietic stem cells can be mobilized either by chemotherapy (in an autologous setting) or by cytokines (in an allogeneic setting). The cells are collected by leukaphoresis and re-infused back into the patient. Many studies are underway to evaluate the difference between this method of transplantation compared to the standard technique of bone marrow infusion.

Maintenance therapy

Maintenance therapy was the rule in the past, when post-remission intensification was not regularily preformed. Study CCG 213 randomized children between maintenance or no-maintenance. It was definitely shown that after an intensive induction and post-remission therapy maintenance therapy was of no benefit. The only large group that still uses maintenance therapy is the BMF-group in Germany (Creutzig et al, 1993).

The therapeutic strategies outlined above apply to the majority of children who develop AML. However, the two following groups of patients need to be given an additional comment.

Down syndrome and acute myelogenous leukaemia

Down syndrome (DS) is associated with a more than 10 times increased incidence of leukaemia. In our Nordic studies we were puzzled by the fact that a high proportion of the patients in our AML-registry turned out to have DS (Slørdahl et al, 1992, 1993). Out of the first 236 children, 32 had DS (10 boys and 22 girls). Their age distribution was strikingly different from normal children since 30 of the 32 were between 14 and 31 months of age at diagnosis. Nineteen had a myelodysplastic syndrome of 2 to 9 months duration prior to the development of leukaemia, and the majority of the leukaemias were classified as M7 (Slørdahl et al, 1992, 1993).

This high frequency is strikingly different from that reported elsewhere (see earlier). Most surprisingly, our children with DS and AML had a very good prognosis if given adequate therapy. This has also been observed in a POG study recently reported by Ravindranath et al (1992).

Acute promyelocytic leukaemia (M3)

M3 accounts for about 10–15% of children with AML. As described earlier, this disease is characterized by t(15;17) where the breakpoints are on the gene for the nuclear receptor for retinoic acid on chromosome 17 and the PML (promyelocytic leukaemia) locus on chromosome 15. The result of the fusion of these two genes results in the synthesis of a fusion transcript which generates a disease-specific fusion protein that in some way is involved in carcinogenesis (reviewed by Warrell et al, 1993). In 1988, Chinese scientists reported that induction of complete remission could be achieved in M3 by the use of all-trans retinoic acid (ATRA) as a single agent (Huang et al, 1988). This was quickly verified by French and American groups (Warell et al, 1993). It is indeed almost unbelievable that a vitamin alone can induce a complete remission in a disease like leukaemia. Of course the involvement of the nuclear receptor for retinoic acid has something to do with the sensitivity of the leukaemia for this vitamin, although the molecular details are still unknown.

The great advantage of all-trans retinoic acid (ATRA) therapy is that the well known bleeding complications of M3 are avoided. What is very clear, however, is that the disease is not cured with this therapy alone and that relapse is the rule unless the remission is consolidated with post-remission intensive chemotherapy. A randomized intergroup study in the USA is now exploring whether it is best to induce the remission with ATRA first and then consolidate with high-dose chemotherapy or whether it is better to start with conventional induction chemotherapy.

It is important to note that ATRA toxicity in children is probably more severe than in adults (Mahmoud et al, 1993). Most important is a distinctive respiratory distress fluid overload disorder (the retinoic acid syndrome). In a recent study, 21 of 78 courses of ATRA therapy in adult patients with M3 developed the retinoic acid syndrome and there were six deaths during induction from this complication (Vahdat et al, 1994a). Low-dose chemotherapy may reduce the complication, but more important is that it seems to be related to a subgroup expressing CD13 on the leukaemic cell surface.

The development of ATRA therapy for M3 has raised the question of whether other types of AML can be influenced by vitamin A. In the Nordic group we have conducted a randomized study on the effect of high-dose retinyl palmitate in all subgroups of AML, but this study has not been finished. However, there are case reports on individual patients with AMLs other than M3 who respond to retinoic acid (Griggs et al, 1994). It is interesting to note that a number of children with the juvenile form of chronic myelogenous leukaemia may also respond to retinoids (Castleberry et al, 1994).

Prognostic factors

In ALL, prognostic factors are well described and include high blast counts at diagnosis, the presence of mature B- or T-cell phenotypes, mediastinal mass, organ involvement and CNS disease at diagnosis. Risk-adapted therapy is adopted in almost all ongoing ALL studies.

Such risk-adapted therapy has so far not been commonly adopted in the AML protocols. The only group that has defined risk groups is the BFM group in Germany (Creutzig et al, 1990). In their study, the low-risk group (comprising 37% of all the patients) included FAB-types M1 with Auer rods, M2 with white blood count less than 20 000, all children with M3 and M4 with eosinophilia. In this group the projected survival after the end of induction in study BFM 83 was reported to be 90%. All the other patients comprised the high-risk group with a survival after remission of 42%.

In other cooperative groups risk factors have of course also been analysed, but with somewhat conflicting results. The impact of age is controversial. In most studies, age has not been shown to carry any prognostic significance, although in the Nordic studies we see a somewhat better survival in the younger age group, even when children with Down syndrome are excluded. The effect of blast count at diagnosis is a risk factor in most studies; the only group that found no correlation between high white blood cells at diagnosis and survival is the Nordic group (unpublished observation). The impact of sex has been shown to be statistically significant in the Nordic material, with girls doing significantly better than boys; no other studies have reported sex to be a risk factor. Cytogenetics is probably the most commonly accepted risk criterion; the good prognosis group includes leukaemias with t(8;21), t(15;17) and inversion 16, while bad prognostic indicators include monosomy 5 or 7.

The translocation involving chromosome 11q23 has been mentioned earlier. Translocations involving this band are very common in infants, and in children with a secondary AML after VP-16 or VM-26. The involved gene MLL seems to be very important in prognosis for infants with AML since the projected event-free survival is less than 20% in infants whose leukaemic cells carry such an arrangement as compared with 80% survival for those without such an abnormality (Chen et al, 1993).

In adults the frequency of MLL gene re-arrangements in AML has recently been reported to about 25%. In contrast to the situation in infants, the presence of this re-arrangement did not influence prognosis (Bower et al, 1994).

Some studies indicate that immunophenotyping may also identify subsets of patients with a grave prognosis. It has been shown that expression of CD33 on the leukaemic cell is associated with a poor outcome (Dinndorf et al, 1992) while the presence or absence of CD34 probably makes no difference. Whether or not the leukaemic cell expresses the c-*kit* receptor or not is probably of no prognostic value (Smith et al, 1994b). Multi-drug-resistance has been a topic of great interest and many studies have shown that the presence of multi-drug-resistance p-glycoprotein (p-170) defines a poor prognostic group. However, in a large study recently reported, there was no association between the presence or absence of p-170 and response to therapy (Sievers et al, 1994). It has been reported by a French group (Wattel et al, 1994) that p-53 mutations are associated with short survival.

FUTURE PROSPECTS

When analysing the results of the large, recently published studies, one is struck by the fact that we all are landing at the same level. We all achieve about 80% induction of remission and, regardless of the type of post-remission therapy, it seems that 40–50% of these children will remain in complete remission with an overall event-free survival of between 30 and 40%. Where do we go from here?

There are two reasons for failures: therapy-related mortality and relapse of the disease. Therapy-related morbidity and mortality is very substantial and has to be reduced in order to improve our results. Death from therapy can occur during induction or during remission after intensive chemotherapy or bone marrow transplantation. Death may be from bleeding, from infections or (after allo-BMT) from GVHD. It is not easy to see how these terrible 'side-effects' can be reduced. If we reduce the intensity of therapy we will certainly increase the number of non-responders and the number of patients who will ultimately relapse. The use of growth factors is one area where a lot of studies are in progress. The two most widely used cytokines are G-CSF and GM-CSF. One of the leaders in this field, D. Metcalf, has recently given his perspective on the role of cytokines both in the aetiology of leukaemia and as therapeutic agents in the fight against this disease (Metcalf, 1994a, b). Preliminary results indicate that G-CSF can be given safely to patients with AML and may shorten the period of aplasia, but no convincing role has yet been demonstrated. The use of GM-CSF is dubious since it may more specifically stimulate the leukaemic clone (Estey et al, 1992).

Do we see new and more effective drugs on the horizon? Well, in the first place, we do not yet know the best way of using those drugs that have already been with us for many years. Anthracyclines, such as daunomycin or adriamycin, are used in most studies and are certainly most effective. Recent studies indicate that idarubicin may be even better (Wiernik et al, 1992) but optimal dosages and schedules for the anthracyclines remain to be found. The cardiotoxicity of the anthracyclines is certainly frightening, and much work is ongoing to explore ways of reducing this danger. The correct dosage and timing of the other highly effective drug (Ara-C) is also a topic of debate. Furthermore, what is the role of mitoxantrone, VP-16, amsacrine and all the others that have been tested in a variety of protocols? It is hard to imagine that we will ever find the answer to all the possible questions that may be raised. There has been one new drug which has proved to be effective in childhood AML and that is 2-chlorodeoxyadenosine (2-CDA) (Santana et al, 1992). In a recent study from St Jude, 22 newly diagnosed children were treated with 2-CDA as the only drug during induction, followed by standard therapy (Santana et al, 1994). Six patients (27%) achieved a complete remission, while seven had partial responses. They also found that the drug was effective against cells in the cerebrospinal fluid in four of six children tested. The ultimate outcome of the patients is so far not known. However, a degenerative neuropathic disorder recently described in adults is certainly a frightening side-effect (Vahdat et al, 1994b).

Many leukaemic cells carry the multidrug resistance gene, especially the CD34-positive cells (for review, see Licht et al, 1994). In some studies the presence of this multidrug transporter is associated with poor prognosis. Much work can be expected on the use of drugs that may modify the MDR expression (List et al, 1993), but no conclusions from the few published papers on this topic can be drawn at this point.

The dream of finding a wonder drug that could act by inducing maturation and that has no side-effects is inside us all. In a limited subset of patients this dream has now been realized with the proven effect of retinoic acid in promyelocytic leukaemia (M3). It has been shown beyond doubt that the induction of remission is really through induction of differentiation. Naturally, this has stimulated a lot of research on ATRA and related retinoids (Smith et al, 1992). The retinoid N-(4-hydroxyphenyl) retinamide is an example of a new retinoid that is already being tested in randomized clinical trials (Delia et al, 1995). Other agents have also been shown, in vitro, to induce differentiation—for example, low dosages of cytostatic agents as well as vitamin D analogues. A very potent inhibitor of leukaemic cell growth belonging to the D-vitamin family was recently reported by Elstner et al (1994). It should not be too optimistic to hope for some substance that may also be effective in other larger subgroups of the acute myelogenous leukaemias.

As mentioned earlier, the use of growth factors as therapeutic agents may be one way to combat infections by decreasing the days in aplasia. However, the use of growth factors in synergy with chemotherapy has also been suggested. The theory here is that growth factors may induce leukaemic cells into growth cycle and thereby increase their sensitivity to cytostatic agents. So far this is a field for the clinical investigator where patients should be treated only within a setting of thoroughly planned clinical trials.

It is my opinion that one of the most difficult therapeutic strategies to evaluate is bone marrow transplantation. An allogeneic transplant certainly reduces the risk of relapse, but the procedure is still associated with up to 20% mortality. Long-term suffering from chronic GVHD is a major problem. The use of unrelated donors should certainly be restricted to patients on prospective clinical trials in order to learn as quickly as possible about both the effect and side-effect. The role of autologous transplantation is even more difficult to evaluate, and there are clearly believers and non-believers in the field. A deeper understanding of the immunological mechanisms involved in GVHD (and possibly GVL), the role of purging in the autologous setting and, finally, the role of growth factors will be exciting developments in the years to come.

It has been mentioned repeatedly in this review that the morbidity and even mortality of therapy for AML is considerable (Sullivan et al, 1992; Liesner et al, 1994). With chemotherapy alone the major chronic threat relates to cardiac function, but for children with bone marrow transplantation, especially with total-body irradiation, intellectual, hormonal and fertility problems need to be taken care of. It is important that children that are cured are given a prolonged and comprehensive follow-up.

Acknowledgement

The author is supported by the Norwegian Cancer Society and The Family Blix Legacy for Medical Research. The secretarial assistance of Vigdis Moen Løkken is greatly appreciated.

REFERENCES

Amadori S, Testi AM, Arico M et al (1993) Prospective comparative study of bone marrow transplantation and postremission chemotherapy for childhood acute myelogenous leukaemia. *Journal of Clinical Oncology* **11:** 1046–1054.

Bennett JM, Catovsky D, Daniel MT et al (1985) Proposed revised criteria for the classification of acute myeloid leukaemia. *Annals of Internal Medicine* **103:** 620–629.

Bennett JM, Catovsky D, Daniel MT et al (1991) Proposals for the recognition of minimally differentiated acute myeloid leukaemia (AML-MO). *British Journal of Haematology* **78:** 325–329.

Berman E (1995) Chemotherapy in acute myelogenous leukaemia: high dose, higher expectations? *Journal of Clinical Oncology* **13:** 1–4.

Bower M, Parry P, Carter M et al (1994) Prevalence and clinical correlations of MLL gene rearrangements in AML-M4/5. *Blood* **84:** 3776–3780.

Boulad F & Kernan NA (1993) Treatment of childhood acute nonlymphoblastic leukemia: a review. *Cancer Investigations* **11:** 534–553.

Burnett AK, Goldstone AH, Stevens RF et al (1994) The role of BMT in addition to intensive chemotherapy in AML in first CR: results of the MRC AML-10 trial. *Blood* **84:** 994.

Busca A, Anasetti C, Anderson G et al (1994) Unrelated donor or autologous marrow transplantation for treatment of acute leukaemia. *Blood* **83:** 3077–3084.

Castleberry RP, Emanuel PD, Zuckerman KS et al (1994) A pilot study of isotretinoin in the treatment of juvenile chronic myelogenous leukaemia. *New England Journal of Medicine* **331:** 1680–1684.

Chen CS, Sorensen PH, Domer PH et al (1993) Molecular rearrangements on chromosome 11q23 predominate in infant acute lymphoblastic leukemia and are associated with specific biologic variables and poor outcome. *Blood* **81:** 2386–2393.

Cline MJ (1994) The molecular basis of leukeamia. *New England Journal of Medicine* **330:** 328–336.

Creutzig U, Ritter J & Schellong G (1990) Identification of two risk groups in childhood acute myelogenous leukaemia after therapy intensification in study AML-BFM-83 as compared with study AML-BFM-78. *Blood* **75:** 1932–1940.

Creutzig U, Ritter J, Zimmermann M & Schellong G (1993) Does cranial irradiation reduce the risk for bone marrow relapse in acute myelogenous leukaemia? Unexpected results of the childhood acute myelogenous leukaemia study BFM-87. *Journal of Clinical Oncology* **11:** 279–286.

Delia D, Aiello A, Formelli F et al (1995) Regulation of apoptosis induced by the retinoid N-(4-hydroxyphenyl) retinamide and effect of deregulated bcl-2. *Blood* **85:** 359–367.

Dinndorf PA, Buckley JD, Nesbit ME et al (1992) Expression of myeloid differentiation antigens in acute nonlymphocytic leukaemia: increased concentration of CD33 antigen predicts poor outcome—a report from the Childrens Cancer Study Group. *Medical and Pediatric Oncology* **20:** 192–200.

Downing JR, Head DR, Curcio-Brint AM et al (1993) An AML1/ETO fusion transcript is consistently detected by RNA-based polymerase chain reaction in acute myelogenous leukaemia containing the (8;21) (q22; q22) translocation. *Blood* **81:** 2860–2865.

Elstner E, Lee YY, Hashiya M et al (1994) 1O′, 14-dihydroxy-20-epi-vitamin D_3: an extraordinarily potent inhibitor of leukemic cell growth in vitro. *Blood* **84:** 1960–1967.

Estey E, Thall PF, Kantarjian H et al (1992) Treatment of newly diagnosed acute myelogenous leukaemia with granulocyte-macrophage colony-stimulating factor (GM-CSF) before and during continuous-infusion high-dose Ara-C + daunorubicin: comparison to patients treated without GM-CSF. *Blood* **79:** 2246–2255.

Gale RP (1995) Cord-blood-cell transplantation – a real sleeper? *New England Journal of Medicine* **332:** 392–393.

Giralt SA & Champlin RE (1994) Leukaemia relapse after allogeneic bone marrow transplantation: a review. *Blood* **84:** 3603–3612.

Goldman JM (1994) A special report: bone marrow transplants using volunteer donors—recommendations and requirements for a standardized practice throughout the world—1994 update. *Blood* **84:** 2833–2839.

Griggs JJ, Henley SE & Rowe JM (1994) Treatment of refractory undifferentiated acute myelogenous leukaemia with all-trans-retinoic acid. *American Journal of Hematology* **45:** 177–180.

Gu T, Nakamura T, Alder H et al (1992) The t(4;11) chromosome translocation of human acute leukaemias fuses the ALL-1 gene, related to drosophila trithorax, to the AF-4 gene. *Cell* **71:** 701–708.

Hasle H (1994) Myelodysplastic syndromes in childhood—classification, epidemiology, and treatment. *Leukaemia and Lymphoma* **13:** 11–26.

Huang ME, Ye YC, Chen SR et al (1988) Use of all-trans retinoic acid in the treatment of acute promyelocytic leukaemia. *Blood* **72:** 567–572.

Imamura J, Miyoshi I & Koeffler HP (1994) p53 in hematologic malignancies. *Blood* **84:** 2412–2421.

Inoue K, Sugiyama H, Ogawa H et al (1994) WT1 as a new prognostic factor and a new marker for the detection of minimal residual disease in acute leukaemia. *Blood* **84:** 3071–3079.

Licht T, Pastan I, Gottesman M & Herrmann F (1994) P-glycoprotein-mediated multidrug resistance in normal and neoplastic hematopoietic cells (Review). *Annals of Hematology* **69:** 159–171.

Lie SO (1989) Acute myelogenous leukaemia in children. *European Journal of Pediatrics* **148:** 382–388.

Lie SO & Gustafsson G (1992) Progress in the treatment of childhood leukaemias. *Annals of Medicine* **24:** 319–323.

Lie SO & Slørdahl S (1985) High-dose cytosine arabinoside in the treatment of childhood malignancies. *Seminars in Oncology* **12:** 160–165.

Lie SO, Berglund G, Gustafsson G et al (1990) High-dose Ara-C as a single-agent consolidation therapy in childhood acute myelogenous leukaemia. *Haematology and Blood Transfusion* **33:** 215–221.

Lie SO, Gustafsson G, Jonmundsson G et al (1992) A population based study of children with AML in the five Nordic countries. Treatment results and risk factors before and after intensification of the protocol. *Medical and Pediatric Oncology* **20:** 386.

Liesner RJ, Leiper AD, Hann IM & Chessells JM (1994) Late effects of intensive treatment for acute myeloid leukemias and myelodysplasia in childhood. *Journal of Clinical Oncology* **12:** 916–924.

List AF, Spier C, Greer J et al (1993) Phase I/II trial of cyclosporine as a chemotherapy-resistance modifier in acute leukemia. *Journal of Clinical Oncology* **11:** 1652–1660.

Löwenberg B (1995) Post-remission treatment of acute myelogenous leukaemia. *New England Journal of Medicine* **332:** 260–262.

Ludwig W-D, Raghavachar A & Thiel E (1994) Immunophenotypic classification of acute lymphoblastic leukaemia. *Baillière's Clinical Haematology* **7:** 235–262.

Mahmoud HH, Hurwitz CA, Roberts WM et al (1993) Tretinoin toxicity in children with acute promyelocytic leukaemia. *Lancet* **342:** 1394–1395.

Maseki N, Miyoshi H, Shimizu K et al (1993) The 8;21 chromosome translocation in acute myeloid leukaemia is always detectable by molecular analysis using AML1. *Blood* **81:** 1573–1579.

Mayer RJ, Davis RB, Shiffer CA et al (1994) Intensive postremission chemotherapy in adults with acute myeloid leukaemia. *New England Journal of Medicine* **331:** 886–901.

Metcalf D (1994a) Hemopoietic regulators and leukaemia development: a personal perspective. *Advances in Cancer Research* **63:** 41–91.

Metcalf D (1994b) Thrombopoietin—at last. *Nature* **369:** 519–520.

Neglia JP & Robison LL (1988) Epidemiology of the childhood acute leukaemias. *Pediatric Clinics of North America* **35:** 674–692.

Nesbit ME, Buckley JD, Feig SA et al (1994) Chemotherapy for induction of remission of childhood acute myeloid leukaemia followed by marrow transplantation or multiagent chemotherapy: a report from the Childrens Cancer Group. *Journal of Clinical Oncology* **12:** 127–135.

Novakovic B (1994) US childhood cancer survival, 1973–1987. *Medical and Pediatric Oncology* **23:** 480–486.

Nucifora G, Birn DJ, Erickson P et al (1993) Detection of DNA rearrangements in the AML1 and ETO loci and of an AML1/ETO fusion mRNA in patients with t(8;21) acute myeloid leukaemia. *Blood* **81:** 883–888.

Phillips M, Richards S & Chessells J (1991) Acute myeloid leukaemia in childhood: the costs and benefits of intensive treatment. *British Journal of Haematology* **77:** 473–477.

Ravindranath Y & Schultz KR (1994) Acute myeloid leukaemias. In Pochedly C (ed.) *Neoplastic Diseases of Childhood*, vol 1, pp 519–540. Chur, Switzerland: Harwood Academic Publishers.

Ravindranath Y, Steuber CP, Krischer J et al (1991) High-dose cytarabine for intensification of early therapy of childhood acute myeloid leukaemia: a Pediatric Oncology Group Study. *Journal of Clinical Oncology* **9:** 572–580.

Ravindranath Y, Abella E, Krischer J & Weinstein H (1992) Superior outcome in Down's syndrome (DS) children with acute myeloid leukaemia (AML): possible link between sensitivity to methotrexate (Mtx) and response to cytosine arabinoside (Ara-C). *Medical and Pediatric Oncology* **20:** 373.

Robison LL, Nesbit ME, Sather HN et al (1984) Down syndrome and acute leukaemia in children: a 10-year retrospective survey from Childrens Cancer Study Group. *Journal of Pediatrics* **105:** 235–242.

Rohatiner A (1994) Myelodysplasia and acute myelogenous leukaemia after myeloablative therapy with autologous stem-cell transplantation. *Journal of Clinical Oncology* **12:** 2521–2523.

Sanders JE (1991) Bone marrow transplantation for pediatric leukemia (review). *Pediatric Annals* **20:** 671–676.

Santana VM, Mirro J Jr, Kearns C et al (1992) 2-chlorodeoxyadenosine produces a high rate of complete hematologic remission in relapsed acute myeloid leukaemia. *Journal of Clinical Oncology* **10:** 364–370.

Santana VM, Hurwitz CA, Blakley RL et al (1994) Complete hematologic remissions induced by 2-chlorodeoxyadenosine in children with newly diagnosed acute myeloid leukaemia. *Blood* **84:** 1237–1242.

Sievers EL, Smith FO, Lee JW et al (1994) Cell surface expression of the multidrug resistance P-glycoprotein (P-170) in pediatric acute myeloid leukaemia fails to define a poor prognostic group. *Blood* **84:** 303a.

Slørdahl SH, Gustafsson G, Jonmundsson G et al (1992) Down's syndrome (DS) and acute myelogenous leukaemia (AML). A population based study in the five Nordic countries. *Medical and Pediatric Oncology* **20:** 373.

Slørdahl SH, Smeland EB, Holte H et al (1993) Leukemic blasts with markers of four cell lineages in Down's syndrome ('megakaryoblastic leukaemia'). *Medical and Pediatric Oncology* **21:** 254–258.

Smith MA, Parkinson DR, Cheson BD & Friedman MA (1992) Retinoids in cancer therapy. *Journal of Clinical Oncology* **10:** 839–864.

Smith MA, Rubinstein L, Ungerleider RS (1994a) Therapy-related acute myeloid leukaemia following treatment with epipodophyllotoxins: estimating the risks. *Medical and Pediatric Oncology* **23:** 86–98.

Smith FO, Broudy VG, Zsebo KM et al (1994b) Cell surface expression of c-kit receptors by childhood acute myeloid leukaemia blasts is not of prognostic value: a report from the Childrens Cancer Group. *Blood* **84:** 847–852

Soutar RL & King DJ (1995) Bone marrow transplantation. *British Medical Journal* **310:** 31–36.

Stevens RF, Hann IM, Burnett AK et al (1994) Improved outcome in paediatric acute myeloid leukaemia: results of the MRC AML 10 trial. *Medical Pediatric Oncology* **23:** 172.

Stiller CA & Eatock EM (1994) Survival from acute non-lymphocytic leukaemia, 1971–88: a population based study. *Archives of Diseases in Childhood* **70:** 219–223.

Sugita K, Furukawa T, Tsuchida M et al (1993) High frequency of etoposide (VP-16)- related secondary leukaemia in children with non-Hodgkin's lymphoma. *American Journal of Pediatric Hematology-Oncology* **15:** 99–104.

Sullivan KM, Mori M, Sanders J et al (1992) Late complications of allogeneic and autologous marrow transplantation (Review). *Bone Marrow Transplantation* **10:** 127–134.

Thirman MJ, Gill HJ, Burnett RC et al (1993) Rearrangement of the MLL gene in acute lymphoblastic and acute myeloid leukaemias with 11q23 chromosomal translocations. *New England Journal of Medicine* **329:** 909–914.

Vahdat L, Maslak P, Miller WH et al (1994a) Early mortality and the retinoic acid syndrome in acute promyelocytic leukaemia: impact of leukocytosis, low-dose chemotherapy, PMN/RAR- isoform, and CD13 expression in patients treated with all-trans retinoic acid. *Blood* **84:** 3843–3849.

Vahdat L, Wong ET, Wile MJ et al (1994b) Therapeutic and neurotoxic effects of 2-chloro-deoxyadenosine in adults with acute myeloid leukemia. *Blood* **84:** 3429–3434.

Vogelsang GB & Hess AD (1994) Graft-versus-host disease: new directions for a persistent problem. *Blood* **84:** 2061–2067.

Warrell RP Jr, Thé H de, Wang ZY & Degos L (1993) Acute promyelocytic leukaemia. *New England Journal of Medicine* **329:** 177–189.

Wattel E, Preudhomme C, Hecquet B et al (1994) p53 mutations are associated with resistance to chemotherapy and short survival in hematologic malignancies. *Blood* **84:** 3148–3157.

Wells RJ, Woods WG, Buckley JD et al (1994) Treatment of newly diagnosed children and adolescents with acute myeloid leukaemia: a Children's Cancer Group Study. *Journal of Clinical Oncology* **12:** 2367–2377.

Wiernik PH, Banks PLC, Case DC Jr et al (1992) Cytarabine plus idarubicin or daunorubucin as induction and consolidation therapy for previously untreated adult patients with acute myeloid leukaemia. *Blood* **79:** 313–319.

Winick NJ, McKenna RW, Shuster JJ et al (1993) Secondary acute myeloid leukaemia in children with acute lymphoblastic leukaemia treated with etoposide. *Journal of Clinical Oncology* **11:** 209–217.

Woods WG, Kobrinsky N, Buckley J et al (1993) Intensively timed induction therapy followed by autologous or allogeneic bone marrow transplantation for children with acute myeloid leukaemia or myelodysplastic syndrome: a Children's Cancer Group pilot study. *Journal of Clinical Oncology* **11:** 1448–1457.

Woods WG, Kobrinsky N, Buckley J et al (1994) Timing intensive induction therapy improves post-remission outcome in acute myeloid leukaemia (AML) irrespective of the use of bone marrow transplantation (BMT). *Blood* **84:** 914.

Zittoun RA, Mandelli F, Willemze R et al (1995) Autologous or allogeneic bone marrow transplantation compared with intensive chemotherapy in acute myelogenous leukaemia. *New England Journal of Medicine* **332:** 217–223.

8

Management of acute lymphoblastic leukaemia

JOHN S. LILLEYMAN
IAN M. HANN

Before treatment became available, children with acute lymphoblastic leukaemia (ALL) had a median survival of less than 3 months (Tivey, 1954). Now, over 70% can achieve normal life expectancy (Rivera et al, 1993). The remarkable story of how this has been accomplished began in 1948 when Farber and colleagues described the first chemotherapy-induced remissions in terminally ill children. The drug used was a folic acid antagonist, aminopterin. It had been developed following the simple observation that folic acid given to children with leukaemia seemed to accelerate the process with the consequent deduction that antagonists might do the reverse.

Other effective drugs soon followed. Corticosteroids and 6-mercaptopurine became available in the early 1950s, with vincristine and asparaginase in the 1960s. Additional drugs now used, such as cytarabine, the anthracyclines and the podophyllins (etoposide and tenopiside), were not developed until the 1970s.

Initially, drugs were given singly and sequentially with the aim of palliation. The next step was the realization that giving them together increased the anti-tumour effect without unacceptable toxicity. However, it was not until the concept of 'total therapy' was developed in the 1960s that the word 'cure' began to appear in the medical literature (Pinkel, 1971). Since then, steady progress has been made through the 1970s and 1980s, as shown in Figure 1.

'Total therapy' is still a valid concept. The idea is to induce remission as quickly as possible, thus improving the patient's basic state of health, and then follow with more aggressive 'consolidation' therapy to reduce tumour burden to a minimum, finishing with a prolonged period of continuing or 'maintenance'-phase treatment. An important component of 'consolidation' is therapy directed at the CNS, because, as more children went into remission, so it became apparent that half or more developed meningeal infiltration after a few months (Evans et al, 1970).

It is helpful to look at the present day management of ALL by dissecting out the following areas for individual consideration: diagnosis and assessment of prognosis, remission induction, consolidation and intensive modules, CNS directed therapy, 'maintenance' treatment, and the management of relapse. Each will be considered in turn.

Baillière's Clinical Paediatrics—
Vol. 3, No. 4, November 1995
ISBN 0–7020–2075–3

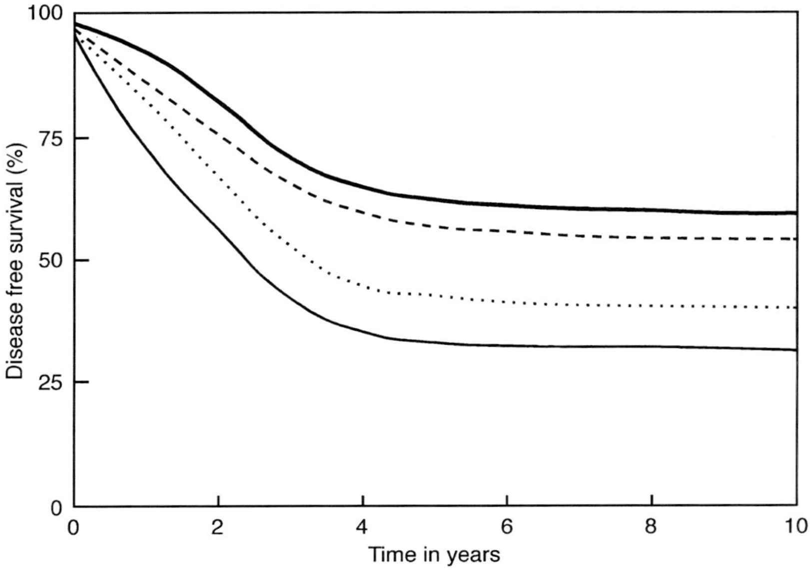

Figure 1. Actuarial disease-free survival in successive United Kingdom Medical Research Council trials for childhood ALL. From the lowest curve, these are for the time periods 1973–1975, 1976–1979, 1979–1985 and 1985–1990. The analysis was carried out on follow-up complete to October 1994. (Courtesy of Dr S. M. Richards, and by permission of the MRC Working Party on Childhood Leukaemia.)

DIAGNOSIS AND PROGNOSIS

Diagnosis

The diagnosis of ALL is usually straightforward. There are two circumstances where difficulties can arise; first, when it is not clear whether the child has leukaemia or not, and second, where it is clear that the child has leukaemia, but it is not clear whether it is ALL or some other type.

The first situation arises most frequently in 'common' ALL where marrow aspiration is difficult and yields poorly cellular material. The marrow may be truly hypocellular as a prodrome to ALL (Melhorn et al, 1970); more commonly, the problem is due to increased marrow fibrosis. Immunological cell typing and cytogenetics may not be much help in such circumstances as there are often insufficient cells for study. If insufficient material for a confident diagnosis is not obtained at the first attempt, a repeat on another occasion is essential.

The second situation arises when it is not clear whether an obvious leukaemia is ALL or some poorly differentiated myeloid variety. This is much less of a problem than it used to be given the current degree of sophistication of cell immunophenotyping and genetic studies, but there are still very occasional cases where immunology can be confusing (showing features of both myeloid and lymphoid cells, or neither) and genetics can be unhelpful. Such examples may be true 'mixed lineage' or undifferentiated leukaemias.

Recognizing that a child has ALL is no longer enough. The disease needs to be classified further on the basis of immunophenotyping and/or genetic analysis, as these features may influence the choice of treatment. As therapy improves, so will the need for more precise definition of ALL and its sub-categories. Currently there are two components that are clinically important in the sub-classification of ALL—the lineage (defined by immunophenotyping) and the blast cell genetics—both cytogenetics and, increasingly, molecular genetics (see Table 1). Currently only a small proportion of children, less than 10%, are selected for other than 'standard' therapy based on such criteria, but that proportion may increase as understanding of the biology of ALL expands.

Table 1. Immunological and genetic sub-categories of childhood ALL.

Lineage	Proportion of total	Immunophenotype	Associated cytogenetic abnormalities[a]	Fusion genes/ deregulation genes
B-precusor	83%	DR+, CD10+/–	Hyperdiploid	–
		CD19+, cIg+/–	Hypodiploid	–
			Near tetraploid	–
			Diploid	–
			t(9;22)[b]	ABL-BCR
			t(4;11)[b]	AF4-MLL
			t(1;19)	PBX1-E2A
			t(11;19)	MLL-ELL
T-cell	15%	CD2+, CD5+, CD7+	t(11;14) (p13;q11)	RBTN2-TCRA
B-Cell[b]	2%	SMIg+	t(8;14)	MYC-IGH
			t(8;22)	MYC-IGL
			t(2;8)	IGK-MYC

[a] Non-random translocations indicated are found in only a proportion of cases, varying from most (e.g. t(8;14) in B-cell ALL) to a small minority (e.g. t(11;14) in T-cell ALL).
[b] These uncommon subtypes are currently selected for other than 'standard' ALL therapy.

Prognosis

As various treatment schedules have been tried, so a varying proportion of children have responded well, and there has been a constant quest to identify them at the outset. This search for prognostic factors has sometimes proved rather confusing, because, of course, treatment itself is the most important prognostic factor making it difficult to assess any others if that aspect is not constant. Nevertheless, it has become apparent that for any child with ALL there are certain features that allow a fairly shrewd estimate of the chances of successful therapy. Some relate to the disease and others to the individual.

Disease characteristics

The diagnostic white cell count is important in predicting outcome (Hardisty and Till, 1968). This has been, and continues to be, a universal finding. The higher the count, the worse the outlook. There is no threshold. The circulating white count is not, however, simply an index of disease stage. Some children with ALL never produce a high count, others always do. Bulky extramedullary disease is also an adverse finding.

Certain genetic abnormalities are associated with unresponsive disease, such as the Philadelphia chromosome (t(9;22)), or t(4;11), and it has been known for some time that B-cell ALL responds poorly to conventional ALL therapy. Better results are obtained if it is treated as a lymphoma (see Chapter 9).

The speed of response to treatment may be related to outcome, and the proportion of morphologically obvious marrow blast cells remaining after the first 14 days can predict the likelihood of subsequent relapse (Eden et al, 1991). The rate of marrow clearance is more likely to be a feature of the type of disease rather than its bulk or extent. Presently, much interest centres around the detection of minimal residual disease using sensitive molecular techniques. Preliminary results suggest that those patients with traces of the original disease left at the end of induction therapy have a higher subsequent relapse rate (Brisco et al, 1994).

Patient characteristics

Age and gender undoubtedly influence the outlook for children with ALL. A third possible factor is compliance.

Age. The matter is complicated as different subtypes of ALL occur with differing frequencies at different ages. For example the t(4;11) ALL described above has a predilection for infancy, and the t(9;22) variety increases in frequency through adolescence to adulthood. However, even taking such factors into account, it appears that, disease for disease, infants below one year of age, and children approaching puberty and beyond, fare worse than the bulk of patients—who fall into the category of children 2–7 years of age. Why this is so is not clear.

Gender. This is also not straightforward, as there are studies reported where there is no difference in outcome between boys and girls (Pui et al, 1991; Niemeyer et al, 1991), but the experience in the United Kingdom and elsewhere has been consistently that boys have a higher relapse rate (Chessells et al, 1995a). The reason is obscure, but does not appear to be due to the fact that T-cell ALL is commoner in boys, or that the testis is a 'sanctuary' site, because prophylactic testicular irradiation does not reduce the male relapse rate (Eden et al, 1990a).

Compliance. The problem is not yet well studied or understood, but it seems that some children do not take their oral chemotherapy reliably during the maintenance phase of treatment, and there is some circumstantial evidence that this may be clinically important (see below).

REMISSION INDUCTION

Vincristine and steroids will induce complete remission in over 80% of children with ALL (Berry et al, 1975). The toxicities of each are not synergistic, and neither drug suppresses bone marrow function. The addition of asparaginase increases the proportion of remitters to over 90% (Ortega et al, 1977), and may also increase the proportion of eventual long survivors. All remission induction regimens for childhood ALL contain these three drugs. Detailed dosages and schedules may differ, but vincristine is usually given weekly for 4–6 weeks, prednisolone daily for 4 weeks, and asparaginase thrice weekly for 3 weeks.

The addition of other agents in the first few days of treatment is more controversial. Cyclophosphamide has been tried without apparent success (Gross et al, 1980), but where remission induction rates are already over 90% it is difficult to see that additional drugs will give a clear advantage in randomized trials with the simple achievement of remission as a measure of outcome.

The question is not just one of remission rates, however, but also one of long-term leukaemia-free survival. The United Kingdom UKALL VIII trial (1980–85) had the addition of two doses of daunorubicin as a randomized variable on the first 2 days of treatment. Although there was no overall difference in remission rates or disease-free survival for those receiving the extra drug, they did show a lower relapse rate. The lack of overall advantage was because there were more deaths in remission in the anthracycline recipients (Eden et al, 1991). Because anthracyclines are widely used in consolidation therapy and in 'intensive' modules, and since there is concern over the cumulative cardiotoxicity the drugs produce, many therapists presently reserve them for use after remission has been achieved. If current trials with cardioprotectant drugs are successful that policy may be reviewed.

The question about drugs used by different therapists for remission induction is confused by semantics to some extent. Over 90% of children will clear their disease (as assessed by marrow cytology) and resume normal or near-normal marrow function within 28 days given just vincristine, steroids and asparaginase. At that point, technically, remission induction is complete. Talk of '8-drug' or '10-drug' induction schedules usually refers to an 8–12 week programme with agents such as 6-mercaptopurine, methotrexate, cytarabine, cyclophosphamide, etoposide, anthracyclines or whatever was being given after the first month. Such post-remission therapy is perhaps best regarded as consolidation or 'early intensification' (see below).

The German BFM collaborative group is unique at present in using a 7-day course of prednisone as a single drug in untreated children and assessing the response to this to stratify them for differing subsequent therapy. The group claims that the strategy identifies about 10% of children who will have > 1000/μ blast cells still circulating in the peripheral blood, and who, by that token, will fare much worse than the rest (Reiter et al, 1994). A conventional induction schedule (with anthracyclines) is then given following the initial week of prednisone.

Complications of remission induction therapy

Drug side-effects are minimal, and most of the problems met during remission induction are disease-related. Asparaginase can cause pancreatitis, encephalitis and disturbances to haemostasis predisposing to thrombosis. Such problems are seen much less commonly than previously, possibly because the product made from *Erwinia* sp is less toxic than that from *Escherichia coli* (Eden et al, 1990b). Vincristine can cause constipation and jaw pain.

Apart from drug side-effects, and bleeding and sepsis provoked by thrombocytopenia and neutropenia, the most important problem is the occasionally fatal *tumour lysis syndrome*. This occurs when there is ultra-rapid tumour breakdown, releasing huge amounts of cell contents into the circulating plasma. Potassium can cause arrhythmias, and urate and phosphate can cause renal failure. Proteolytic enzymes can cause a coagulopathy. Fortunately, the problem is rare, and seen most often in the B-cell leukaemias. It is occasionally seen in other children with very high presenting white cell counts. Simple cell turnover in the pre-treatment phase may be sufficient to compromise renal function before any treatment is started. Renal support may be needed.

To prevent urate nephropathy, all patients should receive allopurinol before being given vincristine and steroids, and should be kept very well hydrated during the first 72 hours of treatment. The management of fever and neutropenia is discussed in Chapter 3 in this volume.

CONSOLIDATION/INTENSIFICATION THERAPY

Initial optimism over the cure rate for ALL in the early 1970s was considerably dampened by a period of about 10 years when little progress was made. The recognition of various prognostic groups served to emphasize how badly some patients were still doing and, although it was possible to define those who had an approximately 50% or better chance of 5-year survival (Secker-Walker et al, 1989), it was clear that minor alterations to therapy made little impact on survival rates.

In the early 1980s a move forward was led by the German BFM group. They administered an 8-week induction/intensification protocol and showed in unrandomized studies that children who received a *further* 6 weeks intensification block did better than historical controls (Riehm et al, 1990). These blocks of chemotherapy contained multiple agents and were given irrespective of blood counts. The idea was to 'hit' the malignant cells with a large dose of drugs in a short period of time. The approach appeared, in unrandomized studies, to produce a dramatic improvement in outcome, and particularly for the highest risk group.

The principle was subsequently examined in randomized trials carried out by the American Children's Cancer Study Group (CCSG) (Tubergen et al, 1993). Patients received either an early intensive 8-week component, a later 6-week component, both, or neither. The trial was based on prognostic groups, and the patients treated were considered to be 'average risk' using criteria derived from results of earlier treatment protocols. (This typifies a major problem with interpretation of treatment results from the 1980s onwards. Despite attempts to reach international agreement on risk groups and trial reporting, this has yet to be achieved so that there is considerable difficulty in comparing trials carried out in different countries.) Patients below 10 years of age appeared to benefit from late intensification therapy. Older children showed a possible benefit from both early and late intensification therapy.

Recently, the BFM physicians have reported the results of their BFM-86 protocol (Reiter et al, 1994). Their 'standard risk' patients (defined on white cell count, liver and spleen size and response to initial steroid therapy) were randomized to receive (or not) a late intensification block at the end of 1 year of therapy. The results showed no benefit for additional treatment, but as only a quarter of the eligible patients were eventually randomized the role of this type of late intensification treatment remains open. The current UK trial (UKALL XI) is exploring the point with a randomized 8-week block at 9 months into maintenance treatment.

Other approaches have included that of the Paediatric Oncology Group (POG) who assessed early intensification therapy using intravenous mercaptopurine and intermediate dose methotrexate (Camitta et al, 1994). This relatively simple two-drug schedule provided further support for the concept of early intensification and suggested that it need not be complicated or contain the more unpleasant antineoplastic drugs. The Boston Dana Faber group has also produced apparently good results with chemotherapy involving repeated doses of doxorubicin and high-dose asparaginase, but there remains a worry over the long-term cardiotoxicity of this regimen (Niemeyer et al, 1991).

The MRC ALL X trial (Chessells et al, 1995b) attempted to find out whether early intensification (after 1 month) or late (after 6 months), or both, benefitted children with all categories of ALL (except B-cell disease). The conclusion was that two courses of intensive therapy are better than one, and that one is better than none. The relative value of early-versus-late therapy was broadly the same. Two intensification blocks produced a 14% improvement in disease-free survival over none. Most importantly, intensification was of benefit to all children, including those at lower risk of treatment failure.

In UKALL X, children with diagnostic white counts over 100×10^9 were eligible for a marrow transplant if a histocompatible sibling donor was available. Of the 198 patients in this white count category, only 34 actually received a marrow transplant. Those 34 had a lower relapse rate than the other 164 but the overall effect on event-free survival was cancelled out by treatment-associated mortality (Chessells et al, 1992).

The precise role of marrow transplantation in first-remission ALL remains controversial. From the UKALL X children it was possible retrospectively to define a group of 8–10% who had an event-free survival of less than 40% at 5 years. A hazard score was thus developed, derived through multivariate analysis of several prognostic factors and using a combination of age, gender and white cell count (Chessells et al, 1995a). This score, rather than a simple white cell count, is currently being used in the present MRC study to select patients to be considered for a matched sibling marrow transplant. It recognizes that young girls with high white cell counts have a relatively good prognosis and excludes them from the transplant option during first remission.

We are thus left with several questions about intensive therapy which are currently being asked in several trials around the world. Current treatment schedules are approaching the limits of tolerance and the idea that even more therapy might be better must be approached with caution. Additional treatment is likely to affect fertility, cardiac function and growth, and increase the risk of second cancers.

CENTRAL NERVOUS SYSTEM-(CNS)-DIRECTED THERAPY

One of the real advances of recent years is the realization that many children with ALL can be treated successfully without cranial radiotherapy, but treatment targeted at the CNS is still extremely important. All patients still remain at risk of relapse in this site and salvage therapy is both toxic and largely unsuccessful. At the present time the most effective and least harmful approach has not been defined.

When considering CNS treatment, it is important to emphasize that the diagnosis of leukaemic infiltration can occasionally be difficult. This is particularly so in asymptomatic patients who are receiving regular intrathecal therapy and who may have a few ambiguous looking leucocytes in their cerebrospinal fluid. One study showed that occasional apparent blasts, without an associated pleocytosis and seen on one or two occasions, are not necessarily associated with an enhanced risk of subsequent overt relapse (Tubergen et al, 1994). One mistake frequently made is to rely upon cell immunophenotyping in borderline cases. Tdt-, CD10- and CD19-positive cells do appear in the CSF of children who do not subsequently relapse, and these markers should be interpreted with great caution.

It is possible to define different risk groups in terms of the probability of CNS relapse, but there is no international consensus on how to do so. The simplest discriminatory factor is the diagnostic white blood cell count. In the current Medical Research Council trial (UKALL XI), a level of 50×10^9 is taken above and below which different therapies are given. All patients receive six doses of intrathecal methotrexate in the early weeks. The higher-risk, higher WBC group are then randomized to receive either 24 Gray cranial radiation or three courses of high-dose methotrexate with folinic acid rescue. The dose used is 6 g/m^2 at which concentration the drug penetrates the CNS. Unirradiated patients also receive subsequent continuing intrathecal methotrexate. The lower-risk group are randomized to receive either high-dose methotrexate or intrathecal methotrexate alone.

The trial aims to explore which therapy achieves the best effect at least cost, particularly in terms of long-term side-effects on intellectual development. The patients are being prospectively assessed using psychometric testing, as presently it is unclear whether high-dose methotrexate is less toxic than cranial irradiation.

Parents frequently find it very puzzling that there is such a heterogeneous approach to CNS therapy, and experience from published studies so far has been difficult to analyse. It has been convincingly shown that a short course of intrathecal methotrexate alone is insufficient to prevent CNS relapse (Ortega et al, 1987) and that, if used as the only CNS therapy, a longer course over at least 2 years is necessary (Littman et al, 1987). Even then it is probably insufficient in the highest risk patients (Blank and Lange, 1981; Cherlow et al, 1993). Whether combined intrathecal therapy with cytarabine, methotrexate and hydrocortisone is superior to methotrexate alone is not known (Pullen et al, 1993).

Recently it has been suggested that the substitution of dexamethasone for prednisolone as part of systemic treatment may offer some protection to the CNS (Jones et al, 1991) and this idea will be tested in the next UK national trial.

'MAINTENANCE' (CONTINUING) CHEMOTHERAPY

The late Professor Tim McElwain once said that the worst way to treat cancer is to trickle in small doses of chemotherapy continuously over a long period of time. In nearly all circumstances he was right, but the one glaring exception is common childhood ALL. Why and how the maintenance phase of chemotherapy works is far less clear than the fact that it does.

Such a statement is not based on randomized studies where maintenance has been compared to no maintenance, but on several empirical observations pointing in the same direction. The evidence has been reviewed by Gale and Butturini (1991). The standard form of maintenance treatment is daily oral 6-mercaptopurine and weekly oral methotrexate. Most therapists also add monthly pulses of intravenous vincristine accompanied by oral steroids. The programme is usually continued for 2 or 3 years.

Attempts to vary this template have produced mixed results. Some studies showed no advantage (or a disadvantage) to adding extra drugs (Aur et al, 1978; Peto et al, 1986) but others indicated that alternative multi-drug cyclical therapy was at least as effective (Sallan et al 1978; Haghbin et al, 1980). More recent reports have indicated that, provided there is some enthusiastic early intensive therapy to consolidate remission, simple 6-mercaptopurine and methotrexate-based maintenance is as good as more complicated and toxic alternatives (Rivera et al, 1991) and a recent overview of all trials examining the role of extra drugs in maintenance at the Second International Collaborative Workshop on Childhood ALL Studies concluded that they appeared to confer little, if any, advantage.

It may be that different sub-types of ALL respond to maintenance therapy differently. It has been suggested that T-cell ALL shows a better response to schedules containing additional treatment with cytarabine and cyclophosphamide whereas non-T ALL shows the reverse (Lauer et al, 1987). It is also now abundantly clear that mature B-cell ALL does not respond to conventional therapy but requires an aggressive 'short sharp shock' high-dose, multidrug approach lasting less than 6 months (Reiter et al, 1992). Presently, though, there is no evidence to suggest that the standard template outlined above is inappropriate for the vast majority of remaining children with B-precursor ALL.

The way 6-mercaptopurine and methotrexate are given is important. Varying the pattern by giving the same doses of the two antimetabolites as concentrated intermittent monthly 5-day pulses rather than the usual daily/weekly therapy produced a clear result in favour of the daily/weekly option in a UK-based randomized trial in the late 1970s (Chessells et al, 1986). The addition of monthly pulses of vincristine and prednisolone adds little to toxicity and is probably of benefit (Bleyer et al, 1991).

Methotrexate

A single oral dose of 20 mg/m^2 once weekly is a small amount, and there is much variability in the serum concentration after such a dose—variability that persists even if the drug is given by intramuscular injection (Pearson et al, 1991). How important this component of therapy might be is not certain. Comparisons of oral versus intramuscular methotrexate during maintenance have not given clear results, though the St Jude group, the Pediatric Oncology Group and the Dana Farber centre all prefer the intramuscular route throughout maintenance (Clavell et al, 1986; Camitta et al, 1989; Rivera et al, 1991).

6-Mercaptopurine

There has been considerable renewed interest in 6-mercaptopurine in recent years (Pinkel, 1992). Its cytotoxic effect, as assessed by myelosuppression, appears to be very variable from patient to patient, and the reasons for this are just beginning to be unravelled. The drug has no intrinsic cytotoxic activity and has to be metabolized to active (thioguanine) nucleotides that interfere with the formation of purines. The metabolic pathways responsible are under genetic control (Lennard et al, 1990).

With the commonly used oral formulation there are many other factors that can potentially interfere with the formation of cytotoxic metabolites, including absorption, trans-membrane transport and, of course, patient compliance. Whatever the reason, it seems that children who form low concentrations of thioguanine nucleotides are at increased risk of later disease relapse (Lilleyman and Lennard, 1994) as are those who do not occasionally show cytopenias as an index of myelosuppression (Dolan et al, 1989).

Boys seem to tolerate higher doses of 6-mercaptopurine than do girls (Hale and Lilleyman, 1991), though so far no gender-based difference in drug metabolism has been recognized, so the reason is not clear. It may reflect a difference in compliance between the sexes.

Whether an alternative thiopurine, 6-thioguanine, might be a better drug to use than 6-mercaptopurine is currently under consideration (Evans and Relling, 1994) and will be tested in the next UK national trial.

Compliance

Most paediatric oncologists have always assumed that children with leukaemia take their prescribed medication reliably, despite growing evidence to the contrary (Davies and Lilleyman, 1995). It seems that a minority of patients fail to comply completely or partially, and that adolescents and some ethnic and social groups may be at special risk. Estimating the extent of the problem is very difficult, but it may be a clinically important factor in over 10% of children in the United Kingdom.

Not only can patients fail to comply, physicians can too, because there is a natural tendency for prescribers to try to avoid treatment-associated morbidity. Such leniency has a price. A Canadian study noted that children persistently prescribed less than the recommended protocol dose of methotrexate (20 mg/m^2 weekly) during maintenance treatment for ALL had a higher relapse rate (Peeters et al, 1988), and conversely, a report from Edinburgh indicated that strict adherence to protocol doses by clinicians produced better results than those from centres where adherence was less strict (Eden et al, 1988). Improved physician compliance is now thought to be a major factor in the impressive improvement in outcome for UK children with ALL that occurred after 1980 (Peto et al, 1986).

Duration of therapy

Several randomized trials over the years have looked at the duration of maintenance therapy, with most comparing times of 18 months, 2 or 3 years. A few smaller studies have looked at 5 years. All that can be concluded is that the best event-free survival is seen in those receiving therapy for more than 18 months and less than 5 years (Nesbit et al, 1983; Riehm et al, 1990; Eden et al, 1991).

Most clinicians currently favour 2 or 3 years, but the choice between these times is finely balanced because, although longer therapy produces fewer late relapses, there are more treatment-related deaths the longer therapy continues. Presently in the United Kingdom all children receive therapy for 100 weeks.

Shared care

The long and drawn out nature of ALL maintenance therapy makes it tedious for patients who have to travel long distances to their nearest treatment centre, particularly as they will be well for most of the time and merely require surveillance with occasional blood-count-driven dosage adjustments of their 6-mercaptopurine and methotrexate. Shared care with district hospitals or clinics is therefore an attractive proposition for some. It is essential, though, for there to be faultless communication between the treatment centre and the shared-care satellite, and for the local service to be staffed by enthusiastic clinicians and nurses familiar with chemotherapy and the management of bone marrow failure.

TREATMENT AFTER RELAPSE

Up to now there has been little hope for the approximately one-third to one-quarter of children who relapse, particularly if this occurs early, while still on treatment. However, universal therapeutic nihilism is being replaced by controversy and uncertainty, indicative of the development of potentially successful new salvage strategies.

Presently it is generally accepted that allogeneic bone marrow transplantation is the treatment of choice for early marrow relapse, but there are three current problems with this approach:

1. Only about a quarter of patients will have a matched sibling donor.
2. The late effects of the preparative regimens (usually total body irradiation and high-dose cyclophosphamide) on the heart, brain, growth, hormones and fertility are considerable.
3. The subsequent relapse rate remains unacceptably high.

The lack of matched donors has led to the development of unrelated donor (UD) marrow transplants. The immediate mortality of this procedure has fallen dramatically in the last few years and it is apparently associated with a lower subsequent relapse rate—a benefit due perhaps to an enhanced graft-versus-leukaemia effect (Cornish et al, 1993). However, UD transplants are still associated with severe early and late toxicity as well as high cost, so their wholesale application is not justified at the present time. Careful evaluation is needed. In the current MRC ALL trial for relapsed patients, those at high risk of failure with conventional salvage therapy and no matched sibling donor are eligible for randomization to receive a UD transplant or intensive chemotherapy.

Attempts to reduce the still-high relapse rate following marrow transplants have been made by using different and even more intensive preparative regimens. There is no convincing evidence at present that this has helped, but alternative approaches such as lower doses of cyclosporin, seeking to enhance the graft-versus-leukaemia effect, encourage further trials (Hunter et al, 1993).

CNS relapse

The best treatment for CNS relapse is not defined. Most centres have now stopped irradiating the spine, as the benefits are dubious and it tends to compromise tolerance of systemic chemotherapy, but for children who have not had cranial radiotherapy and who relapse after 3 years from diagnosis, a 46% chance of event-free survival has been described following remission induction, cranial irradiation and monthly intrathecal drugs (Winick et al, 1993). Children relapsing earlier do less well. Whether marrow transplantation can cure CNS disease is open to debate. Second courses of cranial irradiation within 12–24 months of the first produce a high risk of diffuse encephalopathy.

Testicular relapse

Isolated testicular relapse can be cured with local radiotherapy and intensified chemotherapy if it occurs after 30 months from diagnosis (Henze et al, 1991), but earlier relapses are associated with shorter survival and marrow transplantation should be considered.

Future directions

In view of the expense and toxicity of transplants it is to be hoped that an effective chemotherapy option can be found. Early analyses of intensified chemotherapy relapse schedules look quite encouraging, but there are few effective new drugs on the horizon. Researchers are turning to other approaches such as the potential of agents like interleukin-4 to induce apoptosis or programmed cell death (Manabe et al, 1994).

SUMMARY

Given the best currently available chemotherapy, all but the occasional child with ALL will remit, and about 70% of them will become long-term disease-free survivors. Within that global figure are winners and losers. Around 10% of patients can be recognized prospectively (based on the pattern of age, gender, and diagnostic leucocyte count or on blast cell cytogenetics) who will have a greater than 50% chance of early relapse.

Many unanswered questions about treatment remain. In first-time therapy, both the optimum design and timing of 'intensive' modules of therapy have yet to be defined. The best way to prevent CNS infiltration has not yet been agreed, and even simple matters like the most effective analogue of corticosteroids or thiopurines to use is uncertain. There is also no standardized length of time for the 'maintenance' phase of therapeutic schedules, and the question of patient compliance has not been tackled.

As overall results improve, so it becomes increasingly difficult to make great strides forward, and the law of diminishing returns begins to apply. It is premature, though, to feel complacent about the adequacy of therapy and to concentrate primarily on long-term toxicity. Too many children, between 1 in 4 and 1 in 5, still unpredictably and inexplicably relapse, and salvage therapy for them is still eventually unsuccessful in the majority of cases.

For patients with 'high risk' or recurrent disease there is much work to be done. Neither the best use of marrow transplants nor the best 'conditioning' regimen for them is yet clear, and for patients without histocompatible siblings the risk:benefit ratio and cost effectiveness of using unrelated donors still requires careful evaluation. Intensive chemotherapy schedules as an alternative to marrow transplantation also need to be properly assessed in the context of rigorous multicentre collaborative studies.

Such studies require careful planning, and construction and should be conducted in a limited number of centres under the scrutiny of disinterested statisticians and health economists. It is only through continuing such cooperative efforts that the progress made in the last 40 years is likely to be maintained.

REFERENCES

Aur RJA, Simone JV, Verzosa MS et al (1978) Childhood acute lymphocytic leukemia, Study VIII. *Cancer* **42:** 2123–2134.

Barrett AJ, Horowitz MM, Pollock BH et al (1994) Bone marrow transplants from HLA-identical siblings as compared with chemotherapy for children with acute lymphoblastic leukemia in a second remission. *New England Journal of Medicine* **331:** 1253–1258.

Berry OH, Pullen J, George S et al (1975) Comparison of prednisolone, vincristine, methotrexate and 6-mercaptopurine versus vincristine and prednisone induction therapy in childhood acute leukemia. *Cancer* **36:** 98–102.

Blank J & Lange B (1981) Preleukemia in children. *Journal of Pediatrics* **98:** 565–568.

Bleyer WA, Sather HN, Nickerson HJ et al (1991) Monthly pulses of vincristine and prednisone prevent bone marrow and testicular relapse in low-risk childhood acute lymphoblastic leukemia: a report of the CCG-161 study by the Children's Cancer Study Group. *Journal of Clinical Oncology* **9:** 1012–1021.

Brisco MJ, Condon J, Hughes E et al (1994) Outcome prediction in childhood lymphoblastic leukaemia by molecular quantitation of residual disease at the end of induction. *Lancet* **343:** 196–200.

Camitta B, Leventhal B, Laver S et al (1989) Intermediate dose intravenous methotrexate and mercaptopurine therapy for non-T, non-B acute lymphocytic leukemia of childhood. A Paediatric Oncology Group Study. *Journal of Clinical Oncology* **7:** 1539–1543.

Camitta B, Mahoney D, Leventhal B et al (1994) Intensive intravenous methotrexate and mercaptopurine treatment of higher-risk non-T, non-B acute lymphocytic leukemia: a pediatric oncology group study. *Journal of Clinical Oncology* **12:** 1383–1389.

Cherlow JM, Steinherz PG, Sather HN et al (1993) The role of radiation therapy in the treatment of acute lymphoblastic leukemia with lymphomatous presentation: a report from the Children's Cancer Group. *International Journal of Radiation Oncology Biology and Physiology* **27:** 1001–1009.

Chessells JM, Durrant J, Hardy RM & Richards SM (1986) Medical Research Council Leukaemia Trial—UKALL V: an attempt to reduce the immunosuppressive effects of therapy in childhood acute lymphoblastic leukemia. Report to the Council by the Working Party on Leukaemia in Childhood. *Journal of Clinical Oncology* **4:** 1758–1764.

Chessells JM, Bailey CC, Wheeler K et al (1992) Bone marrow transplantation for high-risk childhood lymphoblastic leukaemia in first remission: experience in MRC UKALL X. *Lancet* **340:** 565–568.

Chessells JM, Richards SM, Bailey CC et al (1995a) Gender and treatment outcome in childhood lymphoblastic leukaemia: report from the MRC UKALL Trials. *British Journal of Haematology* **89:** 364–372.

Chessells JM, Bailey CC & Richards SM (1995b) Intensification of treatment improves survival for all children with lymphoblastic leukaemia: results of MRC UKALL X. *Lancet* **345:** 143–148.

Clavell LA, Gelber RD, Cohen HJ et al (1986) Four agent induction and intensive asparaginase therapy for treatment of childhood acute lymphoblastic leukemia. *New England Journal of Medicine* **315:** 657–663.

Cornish J, Martin A, Pamphilon D & Oakhill A (1993) Effect of HLA-mismatching on the outcome of unrelated donor BMT in children. *British Journal of Haematology* **84 (supplement 1):** 11.

Davies HA & Lilleyman JS (1995) Compliance with oral chemotherapy in childhood lymphoblastic leukaemia. *Cancer Treatment Reviews* **21:** 93–103.

Dolan G, Lilleyman JS & Richards SM (1989) Prognostic importance of myelosuppression during maintenance treatment of lymphoblastic leukaemia. *Archives of Disease in Childhood* **64:** 1231–1234.

Eden OB, Stiller CA & Gerrard MP (1988) Improved survival for childhood acute lymphoblastic leukaemia: possible effect of protocol compliance. *Pediatric Hematology and Oncology* **5:** 83–91.

Eden OB, Lilleyman JS & Richards SM (1990a) Testicular irradiation in childhood lymphoblastic leukaemia. *British Journal of Haematology* **75:** 496–498.

Eden OB, Shaw MP, Lilleyman JS & Richards SM (1990b) Non-randomised study comparing toxicity of *Escherichia coli* and *Erwinia* asparaginase in children with leukaemia. *Medical and Pediatric Oncology* **18:** 497–502.

Eden OB, Lilleyman JS & Richards SM (1991) Results of Medical Research Council Childhood Leukaemia Trial UKALL VIII (Report to the Medical Research Council on behalf of the Working Party on Leukaemia in Childhood). *British Journal of Haematology* **78:** 187–196.

Evans WE & Relling MV (1994) Mercaptopurine vs thioguanine for the treatment of acute lymphoblastic leukemia. *Leukemia Research* **18:** 811–814.

Evans AE, Gilbert ES & Zandstra R (1970) The increasing incidence of central nervous system leukemia in children (Children's Cancer Study Group A). *Cancer* **26:** 404–409.

Farber S, Diamond LK, Mercer RD et al (1948) Temporary remissions in acute leukemia in children produced by folic acid antagonist, 4-aminopteroyl-glutamic acid (aminopterin). *New England Journal of Medicine* **238:** 787–793.

Gale R & Butturini A (1991) Maintenance chemotherapy and cure of childhood lymphoblastic leukaemia. *Lancet* **338:** 1315–1318.

Gross S, Siegel S, Coccia P et al (1980) A toxicity study of cyclophosphamide in combination induction therapy in childhood acute lymphocytic leukemia: a report for the Children's Cancer Study Group. *American Journal of Pediatric Hematology/Oncology* **2:** 321–325.

Haghbin M, Murphy ML, Tan C et al (1980) A long term clinical follow up of children with acute lymphoblastic leukemia treated with intensive chemotherapy regimens. *Cancer* **46:** 241–252.

Hale JP & Lilleyman JS (1991) Importance of 6-mercaptopurine dose in lymphoblastic leukaemia. *Archives of Disease in Childhood* **66:** 462–466.

Hardisty RM & Till M (1968) Acute leukaemia 1959–64. Factors affecting prognosis. *Archives of Disease in Childhood* **43:** 107–115.

Henze G, Fengler R, Hartmann R et al (1991) Six-year experience with a comprehensive approach to the treatment of recurrent childhood acute lymphoblastic leukemia (ALL-REZ BFM 85). A relapse study of the BFM Group. *Blood* **78:** 1166–1172.

Hunter AE, Rogers SY & Russell NH (1993) Low dosage cyclosporin and methotrexate prophylaxis for acute GVHD is associated with a low relative risk of recurrent leukaemia. *British Journal of Haematology* **84 (supplement 1):** 11.

Jones B, Freeman AI, Shuster JJ et al (1991) Lower incidence of meningeal leukaemia when prednisolone is replaced by dexamethasone in the treatment of acute lymphocytic leukemia. *Medical and Pediatric Oncology* **19:** 269–275.

Lauer SJ, Pinkel D, Buchanan G et al (1987) Cytosine arabinoside/cyclophosphamide pulses during continuing therapy for childhood acute lymphoblastic leukaemia. *Cancer* **60:** 2366–2371.

Lennard L, Lilleyman JS, van Loon J & Weinshilboum RM (1990) Genetic variation in response to 6-mercaptopurine for childhood acute lymphoblastic leukaemia. *Lancet* **336:** 225–229.

Lilleyman JS & Lennard L (1994) Mercaptopurine metabolism and risk of relapse in childhood lymphoblastic leukaemia. *Lancet* **343:** 1188–1990.

Littman P, Coccia P, Bleyer WA et al (1987) Central nervous system (CNS) prophylaxis in children with low risk acute lymphoblastic leukemia (ALL). *International Journal of Radiation Oncology Biology Physiology* **13:** 1443–1449.

Manabe A, Coustan-Smith E, Kumagai M-A et al (1994) Interleukin-4 induces programmed cell death (apoptosis) in cases of high-risk acute lymphoblastic leukemia. *Blood* **83:** 1731–1737.

Melhorn DK, Goss S & Newman AJ (1970) Acute childhood leukemia presenting as aplastic anaemia. The response to corticosteroids. *Journal of Pediatrics* **77:** 647–652.

Nesbit ME, Sather HN, Robinson LL et al (1983) Randomized study of 3 years versus 5 years of chemotherapy in childhood acute lymphoblastic leukemia. *Journal of Clinical Oncology* **1:** 308–316.

Niemeyer CM, Reiter A, Riehm H et al (1991) Comparative results of two intensive treatment programs for childhood acute lymphoblastic leukemia: the Berlin–Frankfurt–Münster and Dana-Farber Cancer Institute protocols. *Annals of Oncology* **2:** 745–749.

Ortega JA, Nesbit ME, Donaldson MH et al (1977) L-asparaginase, vincristine and prednisone for induction of first remission in acute lymphocytic leukemia. *Cancer Research* **37:** 535–540.

Ortega JA, Nesbit ME, Sather HN et al (1987) Long-term evaluation of a CNS prophylaxis trial-treatment comparison and outcome after CNS relapse in childhood ALL: a report from the Children's Cancer Study Group. *Journal of Clinical Oncology* **5:** 1646–1654.

Pearson ADJ, Mills S, Amineddine HA et al (1991) The influence of serum methotrexate concentrations and drug dosage on outcome in childhood acute lymphoblastic leukaemia. *British Journal of Cancer* **64:** 169–173.

Peeters M, Koren G, Jakubovicz D & Zipursky A (1988) Physician compliance and relapse rates of acute lymphoblastic leukemia in children. *Clinical Pharmacology Therapeutics* **43:** 228–232.

Peto J, Eden OB, Lilleyman JS & Richards S (1986) Improvement in treatment for children with acute lymphoblastic leukaemia. The Medical Research Council UKALL Trials, 1972–84. Report to the Council by the Working Party on Leukaemia in Childhood. *Lancet* **i:** 408–411.

Pinkel D (1971) Five-year follow-up of 'total therapy' of childhood lymphocytic leukemia. *Journal of American Medical Association* **216:** 648–652.

Pinkel D (1992) Lessons from 20 years of curative therapy of childhood acute leukaemia. *British Journal of Cancer* **65:** 148–153.

Pui C-H, Dodge RK, Look AT et al (1991) Risk of adverse events in children completing treatment for acute lymphoblastic leukemia: St Jude total therapy studies VIII, IX and X. *Journal of Clinical Oncology* **9:** 1341–1347.

Pullen J, Boyett J, Shuster J et al (1993) Extended triple intrathecal chemotherapy trial for prevention of CNS relapse in good-risk and poor-risk patients with B-progenitor acute lymphoblastic leukemia: a Pediatric Oncology Group study. *Journal of Clinical Oncology* **11:** 839–849.

Reiter A, Schrappe M, Ludwig W-D et al (1992) Favourable outcome of B-cell acute lymphoblastic leukemia in childhood: a report of three consecutive studies of the BFM group. *Blood* **80:** 2471–2478.

Reiter A, Schrappe M, Ludwig W-D et al (1994) Chemotherapy in 998 unselected childhood acute lymphoblastic leukemia patients. Results and conclusions of the Multicenter Trial ALL-BFM 86. *Blood* **84:** 3122–3133.

Riehm H, Gadner H, Henze G et al (1990) Results and significance of six randomized trials in four consecutive ALL-BFM studies. *Hematology and Blood Transfusion* **33:** 439–450.

Rivera GK, Raimondi SC, Hancock ML et al (1991) Improved outcome in childhood acute lymphoblastic leukaemia with reinforced early treatment and rotational combination chemotherapy. *Lancet* **337:** 61–66.

Rivera GK, Pinkel D, Simone JV, Hancock ML, Crist WM (1993) Treatment of acute lymphoblastic leukemia: 30 years experience at St Jude Children's Research Hospital. *New England Journal of Medicine* **329:** 1289–1295.

Sallan SE, Camitta BM, Cassady R et al (1978) Intermittent combination chemotherapy with adriamycin for childhood acute lymphoblastic leukemia:clinical results. *Blood* **51:** 425–433.

Secker-Walker LM, Chessells JM, Stewart EL et al (1989) Chromosomes and other prognostic factors in acute lymphoblastic leukaemia: a long term follow up. *British Journal of Haematology* **72:** 336–342.

Tivey H (1954) The natural history of untreated acute leukemia. *Annals New York Academy of Sciences* **60:** 322–358.

Tubergen DG, Gilchrist GS, O'Brien RT et al (1993) Improved outcome with delayed intensification for children with acute lymphoblastic leukemia and intermediate presenting features. A Children's Cancer Group Phase III trial. *Journal of Clinical Oncology* **11:** 527–537.

Tubergen DG, Cullen JW, Boyett JM et al (1994) Blasts in the CSF with a normal cell count do not justify alteration for acute lymphoblastic leukemia in remission: a children's Cancer Group study. *Journal of Clinical Oncology* **12:** 272–278.

Winick NJ, Smith SD, Shuster J et al (1993) Treatment of CNS relapse in children with acute lymphoblastic leukemia: a Pediatric Oncology Group study. *Journal of Clinical Oncology* **11:** 271–278.

9

Management of paediatric lymphomas

CATHERINE PATTE

There are two main categories of lymphomas in childhood which can be considered separately: Hodgkin's disease and non-Hodgkin's lymphoma (NHL). The first category is, above all, a nodal disease and was one of the first curable malignant diseases. It is similar in adults and children, but poses therapeutic problems in children due to long-term radiotherapeutic sequelae. The second category is, above all, a visceral disease which is highly aggressive, and whose catastrophic outcome has recently been completely changed; it will be considered first in this chapter.

NON-HODGKIN'S LYMPHOMA

The term non-Hodgkin's lymphoma (NHL) describes a heterogeneous group of malignant proliferations of lymphoid tissue. In childhood, they differ from those seen in adults by (i) their diffuse, high-grade histology, (ii) the clinical presentation dominated by extranodal disease, rapid tumour growth and dissemination, especially into bone marrow and central nervous system (CNS), and (iii) a catastrophic outcome in a few weeks or months transformed over the past 10 years into a highly curable disease due to a better understanding of the pathological process and better use of intensive chemotherapeutic regimens.

Clinical features

Abdominal tumours

Abdominal tumours are the most frequent. They are of B-cell type, generally Burkitt's. Intussusception leading to the discovery of a small excisable tumour is a rare presentation. The usual clinical picture is a large rapidly growing abdominal mass, or masses, arising from gut or mesentery and often involving other intra-abdominal or retroperitoneal structures and associated with ascites. Laparotomy should be avoided and the diagnosis made by cytological examination of fluid effusion or tumour percutaneous needle biopsy.

Baillière's Clinical Paediatrics—
Vol. 3, No. 4, November 1995
ISBN 0–7020–2075–3

Mediastinal tumours

Mediastinal tumours are typically T-cell lymphoblastic lymphomas. They are revealed by mediastinal compression and/or cervical or axillary lymphadenopathy. Chest X-ray shows a thymic mass often associated with pleural or pericardial effusions. Patients are at high risk of developing respiratory distress and general anaesthesia is contraindicated. Diagnosis should therefore be carried out by cytological examinations of effusions or bone marrow smears. If a tumour biopsy is needed, it should be performed by percutaneous needle biopsy or by mediastinoscopy.

Others sites

Head and neck tumours are the third most common; they generally involve Waldeyer's ring or maxillary and/or mandibular bones. The remaining primary sites are nodes and uncommon sites such as bone, kidney, thyroid, orbit, eyelid, skin and epidural. No particular histology is associated with these sites. Diagnosis is confirmed by tissue biopsy with immunophenotyping.

Clinical particularities of anaplastic large-cell lymphomas (Ki-1+)

This disease (previously called malignant histiocytosis) has some characteristic clinical features: (i) usual node involvement, often painful; (ii) frequent skin involvement, either inflammatory symptoms of the involved nodes or distant macular lesions, or a widespread skin abnormality resembling icthyosis; (iii) frequency of systemic symptoms with fluctuating fever; (iv) waxing and waning evolution in a few cases with episode(s) of spontaneous regression; and (v) the existence of some clinical and pathological forms which appear to shade into features compatible with Hodgkin's disease.

Pretreatment evaluation and staging

NHL is a very fast growing tumour which has thus to be sometimes considered as a therapeutic emergency, particularly where superior vena cava obstruction exists. Once the positive diagnosis has been made, a speedy assessment of classification, staging and general evaluation is mandatory to permit treatment to begin with as little delay as possible.

Diagnosis and classification

The diagnosis can be obtained on biopsy material, including tumour touch preparations, cytological examination of effusion fluids, or bone marrow smears. Immunological data are recommended (preferentially obtained on suspended cells from fresh tumours or on frozen sections, but immunohistochemistry on parafin sections is of value) and also cytogenetic studies. For practical purposes, in order to decide upon appropriate therapy, a tumour must be classified. There are two ways of looking at the three main clinical groups. In the USA, the current classification is based upon the histology picture: small non-cleaved cells (equivalent to Burkitt's), lymphoblastic, and large-cell lymphomas. In Europe the classification is based upon immunology: mature B-cell, non B-cell and Ki-1 + large-cell anaplastic lymphomas. Details of the European classification are as follows:

Mature B-cell lymphoma
- positivity and monoclonality of surface immunologlobulin (Slg)
- histology: Burkitt's, or small non-cleaved cells
- L3 morphology in FAB classification
- t(8;14), t(2;8) or t(8;22)
- abdominal primary

Non-B-cell lymphomas*
- histology: lymphoblastic
- immunology: positivity of T markers (CD1→CD8) or absence of T markers and SIg, but CD10 and CD19 positivity
- L1 or L2 morphology in FAB classification
- focal positivity of acid phosphatase reaction (T-cell varieties)

Anaplastic large-cell lymphomas
- histology
- positivity of CD30 (Ki-1)
- t(2;5).

Staging

The most commonly used classification in children is the St Jude's (or Murphy's) staging system (Murphy, 1980) (Table 1). The traditional boundary between lymphoma and leukaemia has been arbitrarily defined

Table 1. St Jude's staging for childhood non-Hodgkin's lymphoma (NHL).

Stage I	A single tumour (extranodal) or single anatomical area (nodal) with the exclusion of the mediastinum or abdomen
Stage II	A single tumour (extranodal) with regional node involvement Two or more nodal areas on the same side of the diaphragm Two single (extranodal) tumours with or without regional node involvement on the same side of the diaphragm A primary gastrointestinal tract tumour, usually in the ileocoecal area, with or without involvement of associated mesenteric nodes only, grossly completely resected
Stage III	Two single tumours (extranodal) on opposite sides of the diaphragm Two or more nodal areas above and below the diaphragm All the primary intrathoracic tumours (mediastinal, pleural, thymic) All extensive primary intra-abdominal disease, unresectable All paraspinal or epidural tumours, regardless of other tumour site(s)
Stage IV	Any of the above with initial CNS and/or bone marrow involvement

* These lymphomas are mainly T-cell lymphoblastic, but are sometimes 'non-T non-B' (immature B-cell) lymphoblastic lymphomas.

by less or more than 25% blast cells in the bone marrow. CNS involvement is defined by the presence of malignant cells in CSF, intracerebral masses and/or obvious neurological deficits such as cranial nerve palsies or cord compression.

Mandatory staging (which can be done in a few hours) and optional staging procedures are shown in Table 2.

Table 2. Initial work-up for childhood non-Hodgkin's lymphoma (NHL).

Mandatory
Physical examination
Chest and nasopharyngeal X-rays
Abdominal ultrasonography
Two bone marrow aspirations
CSF examination
Complete blood count
LDH, serum electrolytes, BUN, creatinine, uric acid levels.
Optional, depending on clinical circumstances
Bone scan and skeletal survey
Local CT scan (head and neck tumours)
MRI (CNS disease)
Abdominal CT scan (st I or abd st II)

General evaluation

Patients may present with other complications, such as malnutrition, infection, post-surgical problems, respiratory distress and/or metabolic abnormalities. These complications, especially the metabolic ones, may be life-threatening and may need their own management or treatment.

Renal function must be carefully evaluated. Impairment may be due to urinary obstruction by a tumour mass, kidney infiltration by tumour or uric acid nephropathy and requires appropriate treatment, including trans-cutaneous pyelostomy or dialysis.

Tumour lysis syndrome characterized by azotaemia, hyperkalaemia, hyperphosphataemia and hypocalcaemia may be present from the outset or may develop during the first week of treatment. Preventive measures are mandatory, including hyperhydration, alkalinization and allopurinol. Strict monitoring of water and electrolyte balance and prompt adequate management of impairment must occur. This requires expert medical care.

Treatment

Prior to the 1970s, the survival of children with NHL was very poor (Lemerle et al, 1975). Only a few of those with localized disease survived after treatment by surgery and radiotherapy, and none of those with disseminated disease. The introduction of aggressive multi-agent chemotherapy dramatically improved treatment results such that 70 to 90% can now be cured. Surgery and radiotherapy no longer has a place in the treatment of childhood NHL apart from rare circumstances. The key treatment is chemotherapy. Its modalities and intensity have to be adapted to the type and extent of the lymphoma.

B-cell lymphoma

Burkitt's NHL, which represents the majority of B-cell lymphomas, is characterized by a short cell cycle, a high proliferation rate, large tumours, early dissemination, especially to the CNS, and early relapses within 1 year of diagnosis. The general principles of treatment are thus: combinations of drugs delivered in divided doses or by continuous infusion; intensive chemotherapy adapted to the extent of the tumour burden; short intervals between courses ('dosage-intensity'); short total duration of therapy; and CNS directed therapy. Serum LDH level, although non-specific, is a good marker of tumour burden and proliferation rate, and has a prognostic value in many but not all studies.

The three main drugs are: cyclophosphamide, high-dose methotrexate and cytarabine (Djerassi and Kim, 1976; Ziegler, 1977; Sullivan and Ramirez, 1985; Patte et al, 1986a; Gentet et al, 1990). Other important drugs are: vincristine, prednisolone, adriamycin, etoposide (VP16), and ifosfamide. They are delivered in various combinations of short-pulsed courses.

Patients with acute lymphoblastic leukaemia of mature B cells (L3 ALL) share the same characteristics as Burkitt's NHL patients and are included in the same protocols. Lymphomas of large B-cells (centroblastic and immunoblastic) seem to benefit from protocols identical to those used for Burkitt's NHL even though these former patients tend to relapse later.

In Europe, two national groups, from France and Germany, have conducted multicentre studies since 1981 which have resulted in considerable improvements in cure rates.

French LMB protocols. Four consecutive studies (LMB 81, 84, 86, 89) were conducted by the SFOP group (French Paediatric Oncology Society) (Patte et al, 1986b, 1990, 1991, 1992b).

The general scheme of the protocol was the same in the different studies:

1. Induction phase with a low dose of vincristine, cyclophosphamide and prednisone (COP course) which generally induces a good tumour reduction and allows time to deal with metabolic and general problems during a period of time free from bone marrow aplasia.
2. Two further induction courses based on fractionated high-dose cyclophosphamide and high-dose methotrexate in association with prednisone, vincristine and doxorubicin (COPAD M courses).
3. Two consolidation courses based on cytarabine by continuous infusion.
4. Continuation therapy with monthly courses including the same drugs as used in induction and consolidation but at lower dose. The duration of this phase has been progressively reduced with consecutive studies.
5. CNS-directed therapy based on high-dose methotrexate (3 g/m^2 by 3-hour infusion) and intrathecal injections of methotrexate, started early and continued during treatment.

6. CNS treatment by a higher dose of methotrexate (8 g/m^2 by a 4-hour infusion), high-dose aracytine (3 g/m^2 × 4), triple (MTX + ara C + corticosteroids) intrathecal injections and cranial irradiation.

N.B. Local irradiation and surgery are not used.

The duration of treatment was progressively reduced with consecutive studies at the same time there was a reduction in the toxic death rate due partly to the increasing experience of the investigators. Bad prognostic factors have been identified and more intensive treatment applied to these groupings: no tumour response after the first week of treatment, no complete remission (with proven viable residual mass) (Helardot et al, 1989) after the third course of treatment (Philip et al, 1988) and CNS involvement.

In the current study, the LMB 89 protocol, patients are classified in three risk groups which receive treatment of increasing intensity (Patte et al, 1992b). The analysis of the first 343 patients included between July 1989 and September 1993 shows an overall survival of 93% ±2% and an event-free survival (EFS) of 91% ±2%.

The EFS by stage is: 94% ±8% for 70 stages I + II, 91% ±4% for 160 stages III, 88.5% ±11% for 35 stages IV, and 90% ±6% for 78 L3-ALL. The EFS of patients with initial CNS involvement is 81%. The LDH level is no longer of prognostic value.

In the next study the plan is to try to reduce therapy dosage, especially of cyclophosphamide (to avoid sterility in boys; Aubier et al, 1989), and its duration, and to remove cranial irradiation in patients with initial CNS involvement.

BFM protocol. Throughout the four consecutive BFM studies (81, 83, 86, 90) treatment intensity was progressively increased, treatment duration reduced and CNS irradiation withdrawn (Reiter et al, 1992, 1995). In the current study (BFM 90), treatment is stratified for three risk groups (which differ slightly from those of the French study). It consists of 3, or 6, 5-day courses including dexamethasone, methotrexate 0.5 g/m^2 (or 5 g/m^2 in the higher risk group) by 24 hour infusion and intrathecal injections in each course, and alternating ifosfamide, cytarabine, and etoposide with cyclophosphamide and doxorubicin. Results on the first 214 patients included between April 1990 and December 1992 were the following in February 1993. The estimated EFS at 2 years was 89% ±2% for all patients, and according to risk groups: 92% ±7% (32 patients with resected disease), 99% ±1% (88 patients with extra-abdominal non-resected disease, or abdominal stage III with LDH < 500) and 74% ±6% (94 patients with abdominal stage III and LDH > 500, or with bone marrow and/or CNS involvement) (Reiter et al, 1993).

The most remarkable finding is the increase in EFS from 50 to 80% for patients with stage IV B-NHL and mature B-cell ALL (study 86) and those with abdominal st III and LDH > 500 (study 90) when methotrexate was increased from 0.5 to 5 g/m^2 (Reiter et al, 1992, 1993).

UKCCSG studies. In the UKCCSG (United Kingdom Cancer Children Study Group) NHL 86 protocol for advanced-stage diseases, next to a standard regimen, a more extensive regimen called MACHO, with HD MTX and HD Ara-C, was recommended for the higher risk patients: bulky disease with multi-organ involvement, CNS involvement, L3 ALL. This resulted in an EFS of 73, 50 and 64% in stage III, IV and L3-ALL patients respectively (Hann et al, 1990; Pinkerton et al, 1991).

After 1990, the LMB scheme was used with results similar to those of the French study in stages III patients, but lower in stage IV and ALL patients (Pinkerton et al, 1993). The reason for this difference is not yet known.

Other protocols. The third largest series on Burkitt's is the POGs series (Brecher et al, 1992; Bowman et al, 1992). Currently, this group is testing the value of HD ara-C and Ifo-VP16 in advanced stages.

The other publications concerned smaller numbers of patients and were generally from one institution (Schween et al, 1991; Gasparini et al, 1993; Magrath et al, 1993).

Non B-cell lymphomas

This concerns mainly T-cell lymphoblastic lymphomas. The most successful treatments are identical or similar to those of high-risk lymphoblastic leukaemia. The two main ones are the LSA2L2 protocol described by Wollner in New York (and those derived from it) (Wollner et al, 1979), and the LAL-BFM protocol initiated by Riehm in Germany.

Treatment has to be intensive, semicontinuous, for 1 to 2 years, including CNS prophylaxis and numerous drugs (corticosteroids, vincristine, cyclophosphamide, anthracyclines, methotrexate, epipodophyllotoxins, cytosine-arabinoside, asparaginase, 6-mercaptopurine and/or 6-thioguanine).

The results of treatment show an EFS of about 75% with some late relapses (Vecchi et al, 1981; Anderson et al, 1983, 1993; Sullivan et al, 1985; Saha et al, 1995; Patte et al, 1991, 1992; Eden et al, 1992; Bergeron et al, 1993; Katz et al, 1993; Reiter et al, 1995). No other improvement has been obtained in recent years, although therapy has been increased. This is striking in the BFM studies where results in 1993 were similar to those obtained with the protocol 1975 (Schrappe et al, 1993).

Ki-1-positive anaplastic large-cell lymphomas

This disease is rare, and thus even the largest study groups can include only about 10 patients/year which makes the design of trials very difficult. In the USA, these lymphomas have been included in the same protocols as the other large-cell lymphomas and have not been considered as a special entity, making it difficult to be sure how to manage these specific patients. In Europe, they have been considered to be a specific entity. Although treated with either 'B-cell-like' or 'T-cell like' protocols the overall survival rate has been similar at 70–80% (Brugières et al, 1989; Vecchi et al, 1993; Reiter et al, 1994). Event-free survival is often lower, indicating that relapses can be salvaged, particularly if the first-line treatment was not very intensive. Many questions remain. Is it one or several diseases? What are the prognostic factors? (It seems that cutaneous involvement and possibly mediastinal (or lung) involvement are indicators of a bad prognosis.) Which is the best 'type' of treatment?

Bone marrow transplantation

What is the place for high-dose chemotherapy followed by bone marrow transplantation?

Because of a high cure rate, there is no indication for the use of this procedure in patients during their first complete remission. Neither is there an indication for its use in patients in continuing relapse. However, it should be considered for patients who achieved only a partial remission and for patients who relapse and responded to second-line chemotherapy (Hartmann et al, 1984; Philip et al, 1988; Avet-Loiseau et al, 1991; Ebell et al, 1993; Philip et al, 1993).

Conclusion concerning NHL

Dramatic improvements have been obtained in the past 10 years in cure rates for children with NHL, particularly of the B-cell type. This is due in great part to prospective well conducted national multicentre studies, including a large number of patients. These have ensured an increase in knowledge about the diseases and the identification of new prognostic factors, and have allowed a more rational (cost-effective) approach to the use of chemotherapy.

HODGKIN'S DISEASE

Hodgkin's disease has a bimodal age incidence with one peak in young adults at 15–30 years, and the second at 45–55 years. Paediatric cases represent the beginning of the first peak and explain the increased incidence with advancing age through childhood. The disease is uncommon before the age of 5 years. However, in developing countries it occurs more frequently among children less than 10 years of age.

Clinical presentation—diagnosis

Painless cervical lymphadenopathy is the most frequent symptom (80%). 'B' symptoms (presence of unexplained fever, night sweats, unexplained loss of 10% of body weight in the preceding 6 months), although present in about one-third of the patients, are rarely the reason for consultation and their existence must be ascertained by direct questioning.

An unequivocal diagnosis of Hodgkin's disease is necessary and is made possible only by obtaining adequate tissue samples by an open surgical nodal biopsy.

Staging

Correct staging is necessary at diagnosis as treatment is tailored to the extent of the disease.

Initial physical examination. This includes careful evaluation of all nodal areas, liver, spleen and Waldeyer's ring. Doubtful nodes should be explored by cytology or biopsy if their positivity would change stage and/or therapy.

Mediastinal involvement. Although mostly asymptomatic, it is present in about 60% of the cases. Chest X-rays usually allow its diagnosis, but thoracic CT scan is necessary to define its extent and to recognize lymphatic spread to the diaphragmatic region and extralymphatic extension to pericardium, pleura or lung.

Retroperitoneal and abdominal involvement. The most efficacious way of assessing such involvement has been the subject of numerous discussions and has evolved as imaging procedures have improved.

Laparotomy is a major surgical procedure with up to 10% late post-operative complications, mainly intestinal obstruction or fatal post-splenectomy sepsis. Its use in children has largely been abandoned. It might be indicated if treatment by radiation alone were to be considered, but this option is very uncommon in children.

Lymphangiography used to be the 'gold standard' because it can show lymphomatous infiltration in normal size nodes. However, it requires an expert operator and general anaesthesia for young children. Recent studies show that a combination of CT scan and ultrasound can now be used to study disease involvement below the diaphragm.

Bone marrow. They are recommended only in cases of advanced disease, systemic symptoms, abnormal blood count or local bone involvement.

Table 3 summarizes the recommended diagnosis investigations, following which the stage can be assessed using the Ann Arbor classification (Table 4).

Treatment

Appropriate treatment depends both on a definition of the extent of the disease and the age of the patient. Despite similarities of the disease in adults and children, sequelae of therapy, especially of radiotherapy, are of paramount importance in children. Much progress has been made in reducing treatment and its consequent toxicity and sequelae without jeopardizing a high cure rate. However, identification of the optimal therapeutic regimens is still the subject of debate.

Table 3. Recommendations for diagnostic investigation of children with Hodgkin's disease.

Mandatory procedures
Surgical biopsy reviewed by pathologist
History with special attention to fever, sweating and weight loss
Physical examination with cytology or biopsy of doubful nodes
Complete blood count and erythrocyte sedimentation rate
Chest X-ray (postero-anterior and lateral views)
Abdominal CT scan and ultrasound
Procedures required under certain conditions
Chest CT scan if mediastinal, hilar or pulmonary involvement is present or suspected
Post-nasal space X-ray if cervical nodes are involved
Bone marrow biopsy if systemic symptoms are associated with stage II–IV
Liver biopsy if hepatomegaly is homogeneous
Radioisotopic bone scan if stage IV
Pleural cytology if there is a pleural effusion
Research procedures
Mediastinal gallium-67 scan
Mediastinal magnetic resonance imaging
Interleukin-2 receptor and CD8 serum levels

Table 4. Hodgkin's disease: Ann Arbor staging classification.

Stage I	Involvement of a single lymph node region (I) or a single extralymphatic organ or site (IE)
Stage II	Involvement of two or more lymph node regions on the same side of the diaphragm (II) or solitary involvement of an extralymphatic organ or site and of one or more lymph node regions on the same side of the diaphragm (IIE)
Stage III	Involvement of lymph node regions on both sides of the diaphragm (III) which may be accompanied by localized involvement of extralymphatic organ or site (IIIE) or by involvement of the spleen (III S) or both (III SE)
Stage IV	Diffuse or disseminated involvement of one or more extralymphatic organs or tissues with or without associated lymph node enlargement

Radiotherapy

Kaplan showed in 1970 that the optimal radiotherapy dose needed to cure Hodgkin's lymphoma was 40 to 44 Gy. 'Extended field' radiotherapy treats the involved lymph node chain and the apparently uninvolved adjacent lymphatic regions, whereas 'involved fields' radiotherapy was restricted to the involved lymph node chains.

With long follow-up of the first cured patients and their increasing number, the late effects of high-dose radiotherapy (i.e. 40–45 Gy) are now well known. They correlate closely to the dose, the irradiated fields and, moreover, the age at time of treatment, as the severity of late effects has been inversely proportional to age. Radiation induces soft-tissue and skeletal growth impairment resulting, for example, in cases of supra-diaphragmatic node radiation ('mantle radiation') in a thin chin and neck, a narrow chest with short clavicles and upper spinal kyphosis.

Cervical irradiation induces thyroid dysfunction in two-thirds of patients, and is associated with a high TSH level, but generally a normal free thyroxine. Thyroid replacement therapy is necessary in patients with low levels of thyroxine (20% of the cases), but whether or not it should it be given in the more common patient with normal levels is debatable. In favour of such early intervention would be animal studies showing that chronic stimulation of thyroid by high levels of TSH predisposes to thyroid adenoma or carcinoma. However, the incidence of thyroid carcinoma in children is very low in long-term series (Meadows et al, 1989).

High-dose mediastinal irradiation may induce late pleural or pericardial effusion, or constrictive pericarditis (Cosset et al, 1990).

The risk of chronic radiation enteritis with sub-acute obstruction and malabsorption is increased by staging laparotomy and extensive intra-operative investigation. In girls who have to receive pelvic radiation, oophoropexy should be performed in order to protect ovarian function.

Chemotherapy

The MOPP regimen (nitrogen mustard, oncovin, procarbazine, prednisone), first described by Carbone in 1967, resulted in a dramatic improvement in results in patients with advanced disease who were previously not curable (De Vita et al, 1970). However, its effect on germinal cells became a matter for concern. In male adults azoospermia can be observed after three cycles and is always observed after six cycles. When treated before puberty, boys develop normal puberty, but high-level FSH correlating with azoospermy is observed as in adults (Aubier et al, 1989).

Another four-drug combination was developed in 1974 with completely different components: adriamycin, bleomycin, vincristin, and DTIC (ABVD). It appears less toxic on the gonads, with preservation of fertility in most of the men treated as adults (Bonadonna et al, 1989). However, the known pulmonary toxicity of bleomycin and cardiac toxicity of adriamycin (increased by mediastinal irradiation) are also of concern (Cosset et al, 1990).

Secondary neoplasia (leukaemia, non-Hodgkin's lymphoma and solid tumours) is another subject for concern. The actuarial risk is 4% at 10 years and 18% at 20 years (Meadows et al, 1989). Solid tumours are correlated more to radiation since they occur in a previously irradiated area. With leukaemia, there is a strong relationship between the risk and the total dose of alkylating agents.

The significant side-effects of both radiotherapy and chemotherapy have led the various treatment groups to design therapy protocols which utilize their efficacy and minimize their late effects.

Experience with reduction of therapy

The introduction of an effective primary chemotherapy led to a reduction in radiation: radiation fields were reduced to involved fields (Andrieu et al, 1981; Oberlin et al, 1985; Vecchi et al, 1988; Gehan et al, 1990; Hunger et al, 1994) and the dose was reduced from 40–45 Gy to 20 Gy in patients responding to chemotherapy (Jenkin et al, 1982; Donaldson and Link, 1987; Oberlin et al, 1992).

Chemotherapy was also progressively reduced. It was demonstrated that three MOPP cycles were as efficient as six cycles (Oberlin et al, 1985). It was also demonstrated that ABVD could be as efficient as MOPP in localized stages (Fossati-Bellani et al, 1985; Vecchi et al, 1988; Oberlin et al, 1992). However, a German study failed to eliminate procarbazine in the COPP regimen, a variant form of MOPP wherein cyclophosphamide was substituted for the mustard (Brämswig et al, 1990). VP16 was investigated next with a view to replacing procarbazine with a drug which did not have gonadal or other visceral toxicity. It has been incorporated in new regimens as VEBP (vinblastine, etoposide, bleomycin, prednisone) (Oberlin et al, 1990; Landman-Parker et al, 1993) or VEEP (with anthracyclin instead of bleomycin) or OEPA (vinscristine instead of vinblastine) (Schellong et al, 1994) with encouraging results. However, VP16-induced leukaemia has been described (Pui et al, 1991). However, the risk seems to be schedule- and dose-dependent, so that the use of this drug might not be too restricted if certain conditions are fulfilled.

Some attempts have been made to omit radiotherapy completely (Behrendt et al, 1987; Ekert et al, 1988; Martin and Radford, 1989). However, the amount of chemotherapy delivered (generally six cycles with alkylating agents and procarbazine) appears unacceptable because of the production of sterility and the risk of secondary leukaemia.

At the present time, three cycles of chemotherapy (such as the ABVD, VEBP or VEEP regimens) followed by 20 Gy radiation to involved fields can be considered to be one approach to minimal therapy applicable to most of the localized disease patients i.e. ≥ 95% of the total cases.

Treatment of advanced-stage disease

Only 50 to 60% of the patients with stage IV diseases were curable with MOPP or MOPP + ABVD regimens (Oberlin et al, 1992). More intensive treatment based on alkylating agents and procarbazine is needed and justified in view of the bad prognosis of these patients. The good results of the OPPA (oncovin, prednisone, procarbazine, adriamycin) + COPP (cyclophosphamide, oncovin, prednisone, procarbazine) regimen tested on a German series with 81% EFS (Schellong et al, 1987), were reproduced in a European cooperative study of the SIOP (International Society of Pediatric Oncology) (Schellong et al, 1990).

Treatment of resistant and relapsing cases

After the failure of first-line chemotherapy, complete remission can be achieved with second-line chemotherapy with non-cross-resistant drugs in about 50% of cases. However, cure will depend on the addition of curative radiotherapy. High-dose chemotherapy followed by bone marrow rescue showed good results in adults and children (Armitage et al, 1989; Bessa et al, 1993). The subgroups of patients who need such treatment and the best time to do it must be defined.

In conclusion, many studies have been conducted in adults and in children to try to cure most of the patients with localized disease with the least toxic treatment. However, the most cost-effective treatment has yet to be defined. Patients with advanced disease clearly benefit from intensive effective treatment, but we still have to define its precise role. In other patients we have to elucidate how best to tailor treatment to the individual patient, possibly based upon speed of initial response.

SUMMARY

Paediatric lymphomas can be subdivided into two main groups: non-Hodgkin's lymphoma (NHL) and Hodgkin's disease.

NHL arise mainly in the abdomen (B-cell Burkitt's lymphoma) and in the mediastinum (T-cell lymphoblastic lymphoma). They are very aggressive diseases spreading rapidly regionally and to bone marrow and CNS. Their previously catastrophic outcome has been dramatically improved over the past 10 years. B-cell lymphomas have to be treated with intensive short-pulse polychemotherapy with a consequent cure rate reaching 80–90%, whereas T-cell lymphomas have to be treated with intense prolonged semi-continuous polychemotherapy regimens similar to those used for high-risk leukaemias, with a cure rate at 75%. CNS-directed therapy is necessary in both cases and can be achieved with high-dose methotrexate and intrathecal injections without CNS radiotherapy. Hodgkin's disease has been a highly curable disease for more than 20 years, but adverse sequelae of treatment, especially of radiotherapy, are of paramount importance in children. Many current efforts are being made to reduce both radiotherapy and chemotherapy to a 'minimal' treatment without jeopardizing a high cure rate of greater than 90%.

REFERENCES

Anderson JR, Wilson JF, Jenkin DT et al (1983) Childhood non-Hodgkin's lymphoma: Results of a randomized therapeutic trial comparing a 4-drug regimen (COMP) to a 10-drug regimen (LS A2 L2). *New England Journal of Medicine* **308:** 559–565.

Anderson JR, Jenkin RDT, Wilson JF et al (1993) Long term follow-up of patients treated with COMP or LSA2L2 therapy for childhood non-Hodgkin's lymphoma: a report of CCG-551 from the childrens cancer group. *Journal of Clinical Oncology* **11:** 1024–1032.

Andrieu JM, Asselain B, Bayle Ch et al (1981) La séquence polychimiothérapie MOPP-irradiation ganglionnaire sélective dans le traitement de la maladie de Hodgkin, stades cliniques IA-IIIB. *Bulletin du Cancer* **68:** 190–199.

Armitage JO, Barnett MJ, Carella AM et al (1989) Bone marrow transplantation in the treatment of Hodgkin's lymphoma: problems, remaining challenges and future prospects. In Dielh V, Pfreundschuh M, Loeffler M (eds) *New aspects in the Diagnosis and Treatment of Hodgkin's Disease,* pp 1246–1253. Berlin: Springer Verlag.

Aubier F, Flamant F, Brauner R et al (1989) Male gonadal function after chemotherapy for solid tumors in children. *Journal of Clinical Oncology* **7:** 304–309.

Avet-Loiseau H, Hartmann O, Valteau D et al (1991) High-dose chemotherapy containing busulfan followed by bone marrow transplantation in 24 children with refractory or relapsed non-Hodgkin's lymphoma. *Bone Marrow Transplantation* **8:** 465–472.

Behrendt H, Van Bunningen B & Van Leeuwen EF (1987) Treatment of HD in children without radiotherapy. *Cancer* **59:** 1870–1873.

Bergeron C, Patte C, Gentet JC et al (1993) Treatment of childhood lymphoblastic lymphomas. Results of the LMT89 protocol of the SFOP. *Medical and Pediatric Oncology* **21:** 550. Abstract SIOP.

Bessa E, Pacquement H, Hartmann O et al (1993) Long term survival of refractory or relapsed Hodgkin's disease (HD) treated by high dose chemotherapy (HDC) with hematopoietic support. *Medical and Pediatric Oncology* **21:** 552. Abstract SIOP.

Bonadonna G, Valagussa P, Santoro A et al (1989) Hodgkin's disease: the Milan experience with MOPP and AVBD. In Dielh V, Pfreundschuh M, Loeffler M (eds) *New aspects in the Diagnosis and Treatment of Hodgkin's Disease,* pp 169–174. Berlin: Springer Verlag.

Bowman WP, Shuster J, Cook B et al (1992) Improved survival for children with B cell (SIg+) acute lymphoblastic leukemia and stage IV small non-cleaved cell lymphoma. *Proceedings of American Society of Clinical Oncology* **11:** 340. Abstract No. 919.

Brämswig JH, Hörnig-Franz I, Reipenhausen M & Schellong G (1990) The challenge of pediatric Hodgkin's disease: where is the balance between cure and long-term toxicity? *Leukemia and Lymphoma* **3:** 183–193.

Brecher M, Murphy SB, Bowman P et al (1992) Results of Pediatric Oncology Group (POG) 8616: a randomized trial of two forms of therapy for stage III diffuse, small non-cleaved cell lymphoma in children. *Proceedings of the American Society of Clinical Oncology* **11**: 340. Abstract No. 1167.

Brugières L, Caillaud JM, Patte C et al (1989) Malignant histiocytosis: therapeutic results in 27 children treated with a single polychemotherapy regimen. *Medical and Pediatric Oncology* **17:** 193–196.

Cosset JM, Henry-Amar M & Meerwaldt JH (1990) Long-term toxicity of Hodgkin's disease treatment. Abstract of the Fourth International Conference on Malignant Lymphoma, Lugano, 12.

De Vita VT, Serpick A & Carbone PP (1970) Combination chemotherapy in the treatment of advanced HD. *Annals of Internal Medicine* **73:** 881–895.

Djerassi I & Kim JS (1976) Methotrexate and citrovorum rescue in the management of childhood lymphosarcoma and reticulum cell sarcoma (non-Hodgkin's lymphomas) prolonged unmaintained remissions. *Cancer* **38:** 1043.

Donaldson SS & Link MP (1987) Combined modality treatment with low-dose radiation for children with Hodgkin's disease. *Journal of Clinical Oncology* **5:** 742–749.

Ebell W, Reiter A, Bettoni da Cunha et al (1993) Busulfan, Etoposide and Cyclophosphamide (Bu/VP16/Cy) or thiotepa (Bu/VP16/TT) as conditioning regimen for bone marrow transplantation in poor risk B-cell neoplasias of childhood: the BFM strategy. *Medical and Pediatric Oncology* **21:** 536. Abstract SIOP.

Eden O, Hann I, Imeson J et al (1992) Treatment of advanced stage T cell lymphoblastic lymphoma: results of the United Kingdom Children Study Group (UKCCSG) protocol 8503. *British Journal of Haematology* **82:** 310–316.

Ekert H, Waters KD, Smith PJ et al (1988) Treatment with MOPP or ChIVPP chemotherapy only for all stages of childhood Hodgkin's disease. *Journal of Clinical Oncology* **6:** 1845–1850.

Fossati-Bellani F, Gasparini M, Kenda A et al (1985) Limited field and low-dose radiotherapy + ABVD chemotherapy for childhood Hodgkin's disease. Abstract of the XVIIth SIOP meeting, Venice, 323–324.

Gasparini M, Rottoli L, Massimino M et al (1993) Curability of advanced Burkitt's lymphoma in children by intensive short term chemotherapy. *European Journal of Cancer* **29A:** 692–698.

Gehan EA, Sullivan MP, Fuller LM et al (1990) The intergroup HD in children. A study of stages I and II. *Cancer* **65:** 1429–1437.

Gentet JC, Patte C, Quintana E et al (1990) Phase II study of cytarabine and Etoposide in children with refractory or relapsed non-Hodgkin's lymphoma: a study of the French Society of Pediatric Oncology. *Journal of Clinical Oncology* **8:** 661–665.

Hann IM, Eden OB, Barnes J & Pinketon CR, on behalf of the United Kingdom Children's Cancer Study Group (UKCCSG) (1990) 'MACHO' chemotherapy for stage IV B cell lymphoma and B cell acute lymphoblastic leukaemia of childhood. *British Journal of Haematology* **76:** 359–364.

Hartmann O, Pein F, Beaujean F et al (1984) High-dose polychemotherapy with autologous bone marrow transplantation in children with relapsed lymphomas. *Journal of Clinical Oncology* **2:** 979–985.

Helardot PG, Wakim A, Kalifa C et al (1989) The place of surgery in the remission assessment of childhood abdominal malignant non Hodgkin's lymphoma (NHL). *Medical and Pediatric Oncology* **17:** 322. Abstract SIOP.

Hunger SP, Link MP, Donaldson SS (1994) ABVD/MOPP and low-dose involved-field radiotherapy in pediatric Hodgkin's disease: the Stanford experience. *Journal of Clinical Oncology* **12:** 2160–2166.

Jenkin RD, Chan H, Freeman M et al (1982) Hodgkin's disease in children: treatment results with MOPP and low-dose, extended field irradiation. *Cancer Treatment Reports* **66:** 949–959.

Katz JA, Schween M, Amylon M et al (1993) Evaluation of high dose L-asparaginase in treatment of childhood advanced stage lymphoblastic non-Hodgkin's lymphoma: a Pediatric Oncology Group (POG) study. *Medical and Pediatric Oncology* **21:** 550. Abstract SIOP.

Landman-Parker J, Oberlin O, Pacquement H et al (1993) Localized childhood Hodgkin's disease: chemotherapy (CT) regimen with VP16, Bleomycin, Vinblastine and Prednisone (VBVP) before low-dose radiation therapy (RT). Results of the study by the French Society of Pediatric Oncology (SFOP). *Medical and Pediatric Oncology* **21:** 576 (abstract SIOP).

Lemerle M, Gerard-Marchand R, Sancho H et al (1975) Natural history of non-Hodgkin's malignant lymphoma in children. *British Journal of Cancer* **31 (supplement 2):** 324.

Magrath IT, Adde M, Shad A et al (1993) A new short duration chemotherapy protocol for the treatment of small non cleaved cell (SNCC) and large cell (LC) lymphoma. *Proceedings of the American Society of Clinical Oncology* **12:** 385.

Martin J & Radford M (1989) Current practice in Hodgkin's disease. The United Kingdom Children's Cancer Study Group. In Kamps WA, Humphrey GB, Poppema S (eds) *Hodgkin's Disease in Children: Controversies and Current Practice*, pp 263–275. Boston: Kluwer Academic Publishers.

Meadows A, Obringer A, Marrero O et al (1989) Second malignant neoplasms following childhood Hodgkin's disease: treatment and splenectomy as risk factors. *Medical and Pediatric Oncology* **17:** 477–484.

Murphy SB (1980) Classification, staging and results of treatment of childhood non-Hodgkin's lymphoma: dissimilarities from lymphoma in adults. *Seminars in Oncology* **7:** 332–339.

Oberlin O, Boilletot A, Leverger G et al (1985) Clinical staging, primary chemotherapy and involved field radiotherapy in childhood Hodgkin's disease. *European Paediatric Hematology and Oncology* **2:** 65–70.

Oberlin O, Paquement H, Baruchel A et al (1990) Vinblastin, etoposide, bleomycin, prednisone in CS IA-IIA Hodgkin's disease: a pilot study by the French Society of Pediatric Oncology. *Proceedings of American Society of Clinical Oncology* **9:** 1067.

Oberlin O, Leverger G, Paquement H et al (1992) Low dose radiation therapy and reduced chemotherapy in childhood Hodgkin's disease: the experience of the French Society of Pediatric Oncology. *Journal of Clinical Oncology* **10:** 1407–1412.

Patte C, Bernard A, Hartmann O et al (1986a) High dose methotrexate and continuous infusion Ara-C in children's non Hodgkin's lymphoma. *Pediatric Hematology Oncology* **3:** 11–18.

Patte C, Philip T, Rodary C et al (1986b) Improved survival rate in children with stage III and IV B-cell non Hodgkin's lymphoma and leukemia using a multiagent chemotherapy: results of a study of 114 children from the French Pediatric Oncology Society. *Journal of Clinical Oncology* **4:** 1219–1229.

Patte C, Leverger G, Perel Y et al (1990) Updated results of the LMB 86 protocol of the French Pediatric Oncology Society (SFOP) for B-cell non Hodgkin's lymphoma (B-NHL) with CNS involvement (CNS+) and B-ALL. *Medical and Pediatric Oncology* **18:** 397 (abstract SIOP).

Patte C, Philip T, Rodary C et al (1991) High survival rate in advanced stage B-cell lymphomas and leukemias without CNS involvement with a short intensive polychemotherapy. Results of a randomized trial from the French Pediatric Oncology Society (SFOP) on 216 children. *Journal of Clinical Oncology* **9:** 123–132.

Patte C, Kalifa C, Flamant F et al (1992a) Results of the LMT81 protocol, a modified LSA2L2 protocol with high dose methotrexate, on 84 children with non B-cell lymphoma. *Medical and Pediatric Oncology* **20:** 105–113.

Patte C, Michon J, Brouffet E et al (1992b) High survival rate of childhood B-cell lymphoma and leukemia as result of the LMB 89 protocol of the SFOP. *Proceedings of the American Society of Clinical Oncology* **11:** 340. Abstract No. 1164.

Philip T, Hartmann O, Biron P et al (1988) High-dose therapy and autologous bone marrow transplantation in partial remission after first-line induction therapy for diffuse non-Hodgkin's lymphoma. *Journal of Clinical Oncology* **6:** 1118–1124.

Philip T, Hartmann O, Michon J et al (1993) Curability of relapsed childhood B-cell non Hodgkin's lymphoma following intensive first line therapy. *Blood* **81:** 2003–2006.

Pinkerton CR, Hann I, Eden OB et al (1991) Outcome In stage III non-Hodgkin's lymphoma in children (UKCCSG study NHL 86). How much treatment is needed? *British Journal of Cancer* **64:** 583–587.

Pinkerton CR, Gerrard M, Hann I, Eden OB, Carton R (1993) United Kingdom children's cancer study group (UKCCSG) experience with the French SFOP Intensive regimen for advanced B lymphoblastic lymphoma. *Medical Pediatrics and Oncology* **21:** 532. Abstract SIOP.

Pui CH, Ribeiro R, Hancock M et al (1991) Acute myeloid leukemia in children treated with epipodophyllotoxins for acute lymphoblastic leukemia. *New England Journal of Medicine* **325:** 1682–1687.

Reiter A, Schrappe M, Ludwig WD et al (1992) Favorable outcome of B-cell acute lymphoblastic leukemia in childhood: a report of three consecutive studies of the BFM group. *Blood* **80:** 2471–2478.

Reiter A, Schrappe M, Henzler D et al for the BFM group (1993) Risk group definition, treatment strategy and preliminary results for B-cell neoplasias in trial. NHL-BFM 90. *Medical Pediatric and Oncology* **21:** 550 (abstract SIOP).

Reiter A, Schrappe M, Tiemann M et al (1994) Successful treatment strategy for Ki-1 anaplastic large-cell lymphoma of childhood: a prospective analysis of 62 patients enrolled in three consecutive Berlin–Frankfurt–Munster group studies. *Journal of Clinical Oncology* **12:** 899–908.

Reiter A, Schrappe M, Parwaresch R et al (1995) Non-Hodgkin's lymphomas of childhood and adolescence: results of a treatment stratified for biologic subtypes and stage. A report of the Berlin–Frankfurt–Munster Group. *Journal of Clinical Oncology* **13:** 359–372.

Saha V, Eden OB, Hann I et al (1995) Primary extra-thoracic T-cell non-hodgkin's lymphoma of childhood. *Leukemia* **9:** 40–43.

Schellong G, Hörnig I, Brämswig JH et al (1987) Favourable outcome of childhood Stage IV HD with OPPA/COPP chemotherapy and additional radiotherapy. Abstract of the XIXth SIOP meeting, Jerusalem, 132.

Schellong G, Hörnig-Franz I & Müller RP (1990) Preliminary report on the SIOP study on stage IV HD (SIOP HD IV 87). Abstract. *Medical and Pediatric Oncology* **18:** 426.

Schellong G, Brämswig JH, Hörnig-Franz I et al (1994) Hodgkin's disease in children: combined modality treatment for stages IA, IB, and IIA. *Annals of Oncology* **5 (supplement 2):** S113–S115.

Schween MR, Blattner SR, Lynch E et al (1991) HIC-COM: a 2 month intensive chemotherapy regimen for children with stage III and IV Burkitt's lymphoma and B-cell acute lymphoblastic leukemia. *Journal of Clinical Oncology* **9:** 133.

Shrappe M, Reiter A, Brandt A et al (1993) Childhood non-Hodgkin's lymphoma of the non B-cell type: treatment results of three BFM trials. *Medical and Pediatric Oncology* **21:** 531. Abstract SIOP.

Sullivan MP & Ramirez I (1985) Curability of Burkitt's lymphoma with high-dose cyclophosphamide, high-dose methotrexate therapy and intrathecal chemoprophylaxis. *Journal of Clinical Oncology* **3:** 627.

Sullivan MP, Boyett J, Pullen J et al (1985) Pediatric Oncology Goup experience with modified LSA2L2 therapy in 107 children with non-Hodgkin's lymphoma (Burkitt's lymphoma excluded). *Cancer* **55:** 323–363.

Vecchi V, Pression A & Serra L (1981) Non-Hodgkin's lymphoma in children: results of treatment with the modified LSA2-L2 protocol. *Medical and Pediatric Oncology* **9:** 483.

Vecchi V, Comelli A, Meloni G et al (1988) Updated results of protocol MH'83 of the Italian Association of Pediatric Hematology and Oncology for Childhood Hodgkin's disease. Abstract of the International Society of Pediatric Oncology, 155.

Vecchi V, Burnelli R, Pileri S et al (1993) Anaplastic large cell lymphoma (Ki-1+/CD30+) in childhood. *Medical and Pediatric Oncology* **21:** 402–410.

Wollner N, Exelby PR & Lieberman PH (1979) Non-Hodgkin's lymphoma in children: a progress report on the original patients treated with the LSA2-L2 protocol. *Cancer* **44:** 1990.

Ziegler JL (1977) Treatment results of 54 American patients with Burkitt's lymphoma are similar to the African experience. *New England Journal of Medicine* **297:** 75.

Index

Note: Page numbers of article titles are in **bold** type.